Kimitaka Kaga

Central Auditory Pathway Disorders

Kimitaka Kaga

Central Auditory Pathway Disorders

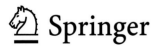 Springer

MW

Kimitaka Kaga, M.D., Ph.D.
Emeritus Professor
The University of Tokyo
Director
National Institute of Sensory Organs
National Tokyo Medical Center
2-5-1 Higashigaoka, Meguro-ku, Tokyo 152-8902, Japan

Library of Congress Control Number: 2009928338

ISBN 978-4-431-26654-9 Springer Tokyo Berlin Heidelberg New York
e-ISBN 978-4-431-26920-5

Springer is a part of Springer Science+Business Media
springer.com

© Springer 2009, Tokyo
Printed in Japan

Typesetting: SNP Best-set Typesetter Ltd., Hong Kong
Printing and binding: Hicom, Japan

Printed on acid-free paper

6/3/10

Preface

This monograph is a collection of my basic and clinical research papers in auditory evoked potentials of my patients with central auditory pathway disorders.

In 1973, it was an epoch-making year in my life when I first became aware of auditory brainstem response (ABR) at a departmental seminar at Teikyo University in 1973, just after I had moved from the Department of Otolaryngology at the University of Tokyo. In the seminar, Professor Tokuro Suzuki, the guest speaker, described ABR to us as a new tool for objective audiometry. The next year, Professor Robert Galambos of the University of California, San Diego, was invited to Teikyo University as a special guest from abroad, and he lectured on auditory neurophysiology and conducted animal experiments of ABRs with us. He ignited a passion in us to study ABRs audiologically and neurologically. Thus inspired, I was convinced that ABRs must be a very useful tool to explore local diagnosis of auditory nerve and brainstem lesions of neurological diseases, coma, and cortical auditory disorders as well as objective audiometry for newborns and infants and for pediatric neurological diseases.

In 1979, a Japan–U.S. seminar on ABRs was planned and conducted by Professor Jun-Ichi Suzuki and Professor Galambos, supported by the Japan Science Council. Since Dr. D.L. Jewett discovered ABR in cats and humans in 1970, several names for this auditory evoked response, including BSR (brainstem response), BAER (brainstem auditory evoked response) and others, had been used in scientific and clinical papers and had confused researchers in this field around the world. At the Japan–U.S. seminar on ABR in 1979, the participants included D.L. Jewett, H. Davis, R. Galambos, J. Buchwald, K. Hecox, A. Starr, T. Picton, J. Stockard. and R. Hink from the United States; and from Japan, T. Suzuki, J-I Suzuki, O. Soda, Y. Shinoda, G. Ichikawa, T. Yagi, K. Kodera and myself. We discussed the proposed names and then voted. The resulting decision was to recommend "auditory brainstem response" (ABR) for use worldwide, and since then the term has come to be used commonly in the field.

At Teikyo University I compared ABRs with temporal bone and brain pathology and conducted animal experiments to explore the origins of ABRs and middle latency responses (MLRs). After moving from Teikyo University to Tokyo University in 1992, I restarted clinical applications of auditory evoked potentials using positron emission tomography (PET) and magnetoencephalography (MEG).

In this book, temporal bone and brain histopathology, computed tomography (CT) and magnetic resonance imaging (MRI) data are presented on many pages in comparison with ABRs in order to reveal lesions in the central auditory pathway. This combined study was made possible through collaboration with the Department of Pathology and the Temporal Bone Laboratory at Teikyo University. I hope that this book will be useful for neurological and neuropsychological diagnosis and neurophysiological studies of the central auditory system from the auditory nerve to the auditory cortex.

I thank Dr. R. Marsh, Ms. H. Miyazaki and Ms. K. Sekiguchi for their unlimited help in publishing this book and for their encouragement.

Kimitaka Kaga, M.D., Ph.D.
Director, National Institute of Sensory Organs
National Tokyo Medical Center
Emeritus Professor, The University of Tokyo
July 2009

Contents

1
Introduction

During the latter half of the 20th century, computed tomography and magnetic resonance imaging (MRI) as well as various evoked potentials have revolutionized the anatomical diagnosis of disorders of the central and peripheral auditory system, and we can expect further advances with such technologies as functional MRI and positron emission tomography. However, auditory evoked potentials have contributed much to our understanding and neurophysiological diagnosis of disorders of the auditory system and still have a very important place which is not revealed by imaging. Defects that are so small as to be invisible to MRI can be detected by evoked potentials. In the case of larger defects, it may be a simple, inexpensive evoked-potential test that raises suspicion of a lesion.

Overview of the Auditory System

Some knowledge of the anatomy and function of the auditory system is necessary for understanding the auditory evoked potentials as they relate to peripheral and central auditory disorders. The major divisions of the ear—outer, middle, inner, and spiral ganglion—are familiar to the reader.

The ascending auditory system is illustrated in Fig. 1 (1). The starting point for subdivision is to define the ascending pathway from ear to cortex. By 1930, it had been shown by studies using the Marchi method for tracing degenerated myelinated fibers that the cochlear nucleus is the first center, the superior olivary complex the second, the inferior colliculus the third, the medial geniculate body the fourth, and the auditory cortex itself the fifth and final center. To stop at this description of the system would be an oversimplification. Several qualifications are necessary, and several issues remain unresolved (1).

Central Auditory Pathway Disorders. K. Kaga
doi: 978-4-431-26920-5_1, © Springer 2009

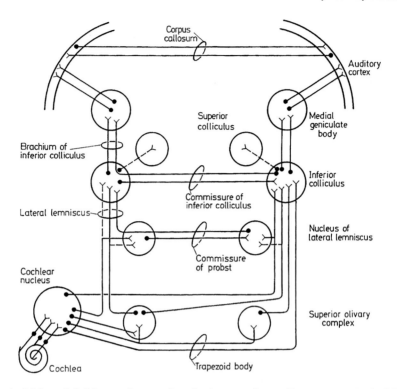

Fig. 1. Major subdivisions and connections in the ascending auditory system. *Dashed lines* represent connections for which experimental evidence is questionable or incomplete. The diagram is intended to summarize anatomical evidence indicating that there are several pathways, in parallel, from the cochlear nucleus to the cortex. The connections for one cochlea only are shown (1)

Development of Auditory Evoked Potentials and Neurotological Application

Auditory evoked potentials (Fig. 2) are classified as electrocochleographic response (EcochG), auditory brainstem response (ABR), middle latency response (MLR), and slow vertex response (SVR). Another potential of interest, even though it is not specific to the auditory system, is the P300 event-related potential. Unlike the other potentials, it is not generated by a simple repetitive stimulus; rather, the P300 is elicited by an oddball paradigm. For example, in the sequence of sounds "pa pa pa BA pa" each sound elicits an SVR, but only the rare stimulus "BA" elicits the P300 (2). Table 1 lists the year in which each evoked potential was first reported in the journal.

The neural generators of these potentials and their audiological and neurological applications for making diagnoses, assessing hearing, and monitoring neural activity have been described in research publications of the author and many other

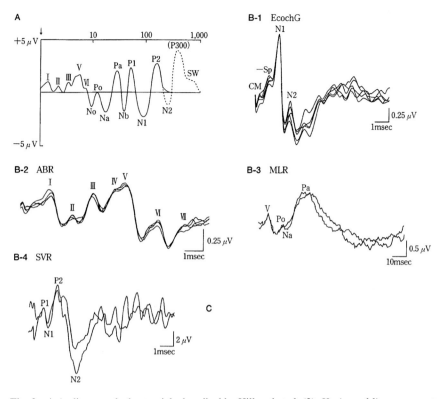

Fig. 2. A Auditory evoked potentials described by Hillyard et al. (2). *Horizontal lines* represent the logarithm scale, and the *vertical line* is the amplitude. *Dotted line* is P300 by infrequent stimuli. **B-1** Electrocochleography. *CM*, microphone potentials; *SP*, summating potentials; *N1, N2*, compound action potentials. **B-2** Auditory brainstem response. Seven positive peaks were named by Jewett et al. (4). **B-3** Middle latency response. The Pa component is an important indicator for the diagnosis. **B-4** Slow vertex response or long latency response, which is the oldest auditory evoked potential, discovered by Davis (6)

investigators. The ECochG is generated from the hair cells in the cochlea, cochlear nerve, and lower brainstem (3). The generators of the ABR are the cochlear nerve and brainstem sources from the cochlear nucleus to the brachium of the inferior colliculus (4).

The electrically recorded middle-latency response (MLR) is generated partly in the auditory cortex but mainly in extensive neural structures in the brain (5); however, it is not appropriate for diagnosing auditory cortex lesions. This is true of cortical responses in general; current flowing to the surface of the brain cannot be localized with surface electrodes. However, the magnetic fields generated by such currents can be localized rather well. The magnetic field generated by the cortical component of the MLR is localized in the auditory cortex. The origins of P1N1P2 components, electrically recorded as a long latency response (SVR), have not been

Table 1. Year of publication for evoked potentials

No.	Year	Author	Name	Journal
1	1930	Berger	Electroencephalography	J Psychol Neural
2	1930	Weber & Bray	Cochlear microphonics	Proc Nat Acad Sci USA
3	1939	Davis	K complex	J Neurophysiol
4	1947	Dawson	Long latency response	J Neurol Neurosurg Psychiatry
5	1958	Geisler	Middle latency response	Science
6	1958	Davis	Summating potential	Ann ORL
7	1963	Kiang	Postauricular response	Q Prog Rep Res Lab Electronics MIT
8	1964	Walter et al.	CNV	Nature
9	1965	Sutton	P300	Science
10	1968	Yoshie et al.	Electrocochleography	Laryngoscope
		Portmann et al.	Electrocochleography	Lev laryngol (Bordeaux)
11	1970	Jewett	Auditory brainstem response	Science
		Sohmer & Feinmesser	Auditory brainstem response	Isr J Med Sci
12	1978	Kemp	Otoacoustic emission	J Acoustic Soc Ann
13	1979	Kemp	DPOAE	Arch Otorhinolaryngol
14	1979	Näätänen et al.	Mismatch negativity	In a book edited by Kimmel, et al.
15	1981	Galambos et al.	40 Hz ASSR	Proc Natl Acad Sci USA
16	1992	Colebatch & Halmagyi	Vestibular myogenic potencials	Neurology
17	2002	Lins, Picton, et al.	Multiple ASSR	J Acoust Soc Am

revealed despite many studies (6). However, the magnetic dipole corresponding to N1 is localized in the auditory cortex, in an area different from that of the magnetic MLR site. The origins of the P300 event-related potential have not been clearly defined (7). The hypothesis of a hippocampal origin has encountered contrasting opinions.

In summary, except for the P300, the auditory evoked potentials have rather well-defined origins and have become valuable tools for assessing auditory function, establishing neurological and neurotological diagnoses, and monitoring neural function. The clinician must not be misled, however, by the ease of recording these potentials. Like any tool, evoked potentials require training and skill in their application. The clinician who wishes to record and analyze evoked potentials must have a thorough understanding of the underlying technical and clinical issues; to attempt their use otherwise is to risk errors and misdiagnoses.

Of all these potentials, it was the identification of the ABR, discovered by Jewett et al. in 1970, that revolutionized the field of objective audiometry and the possibility of brainstem neurodiagnoses (4). Before the introduction of ABR, attempts had been made to apply long-latency responses (LLRs) and ECochG to objective audiometry, but LLRs are variable in infants, and ECochG, in addition to being technically difficult, did not estimate hearing threshold with any precision. In contrast, ABR responses are easily recorded and reliably estimate the hearing level. In neurotology, the ABR has demonstrated a remarkable (but not infallible) ability to detect small acoustic tumors. More than three and a half decades have passed since the discovery of the ABR. During that time, it quickly became the accepted test of auditory function in infants. Instruments incorporating automatic detection of ABRs have become established as the most sensitive and specific devices for universal newborn hearing screening. At present, ABRs are also routinely used in basic hearing research to evaluate small animals' hearing objectively and in clinical medicine to explore brainstem lesions or assess function in such cases as neurological disease, coma, or brain death.

It was the ABR that sparked research in the other auditory evoked potentials. More recently, other new tools to explore inner ear and brain have appeared. Otoacoustic emissions (OAEs) are acoustic signals generated by the outer hair cells in their role in amplifying and tuning vibrations of the basilar membrane (8). The clinically useful tests employ either distortion-product or transient OAEs; the two differ in the manner in which the OAE is elicited and identified. OAEs are indispensable for evaluating cochlear function, especially when diagnosing an auditory neuropathy or auditory nerve disease (9). Magnetic encephalography (MEG) is another new tool for evaluating cortical function. An array of detectors identifies areas of cortical activity (e.g., during an auditory task) with more precision that electroencephalography (EEG) electrodes can. Other new technologies offer the prospect of measuring brain activity without the radiation that positron emission tomography requires (10). Functional MRI measures areas of high blood flow in the brain, and optical topography measures cortical hemoglobin saturation; both offer the prospect of identifying areas of the brain involved in a sensory and cognitive process or that are impaired by disease.

In addition to auditory fields, a new tool to investigate vestibular function has appeared. The vestibular apparatus consists of the semicircular canals, which detect rotation, and the utricle and saccule, which detect linear acceleration and gravity. It has long been possible to assess the left and right semicircular canals separately but not the other receptors. The vestibular myogenic potential (VEMP) measures a reflex that travels from the saccule through the sacculoinferior vestibular nerve and vestibular nucleus to the sternocleid muscles (11). VEMP offers the prospect of side-specific evaluation of the saccule and its projections.

References

1. Neff WD, Diamond IT, Casseday JH (1975) Behavioral studies of auditory discrimination: central nervous system. In: Keidel WD, Neff WD (eds) Auditory system physiology (CNS) behavioral studies psychoacoustics. Springer-Verlag, Berlin, pp 309–400
2. Hillyard SA, Simpson GV, Woods DL, et al (1984) Event-related brain potential and selective attention to different modalities in cortical integration. In: Reinso-Suarez F and Ajmone-Marsan C (eds) Cortical Integration. Raven Press, New York, pp 395–414
3. Yoshie N, Ohashi T, Suzuki T (1967) Non-surgical recording of auditory action potential in man. Laryngoscope 77:76–85
4. Jewett DL, Romano MN, Williston JS (1970) Human auditory evoked potentials: possible brainstem components detected on the scalp. Science 167:1517–1518

5. Geisler CD, Frichkopf LS, Rosenblith WA (1958) Extracranial response to acoustic clicks in man. Science 128:1210–1211
6. Davis PA (1939) Effects of acoustic stimuli on the waking human brain. J Neurophysiol 2:494–499
7. Sutton S, Braren M, Zubin J, et al (1967) Information delivery and the sensory evoked potential. Science 155:1436–1439
8. Kemp DT (1978) Stimulated acoustic emissions from within the human auditory system. J Acoust Soc Am 64:1386–1391
9. Kaga K, Nakamura M, Shinogami M, et al (1996) Auditory nerve disease of both ears revealed by auditory brainstem response, electrocochleography and otoacoustic emissions. Scand Audiol 25:233–238
10. Makela JP, Hari R, Valanne L, et al (1991) Auditory evoked magnetic fields after ischemic lesions. Ann Neurol 30:76–82
11. Colebatch JG, Halmagyi GM (1992) Vestibular evoked potentials in human neck muscles before and after unilateral vestibular deafferentation. Neurology 42:1635–1636

2
Origins of Evoked Potentials

If evoked potentials are to be of any value in the diagnosis of central lesions, it is necessary to identify the anatomical site that generates the potential. This task is made more difficult because many responses have multiple generators. For example, a particular wave in the auditory brainstem response (ABR) might reflect activity of fourth-order neurons, but there may be fourth-order neurons originating from several sites within the brainstem, ipsilateral and contralateral to the ear being stimulated. There are other complexities as well. Although animal studies are of great value, one cannot be sure that the generators in animals are identical to those in humans. Maturational effects must also be considered in the pediatric population. For example, the middle latency response, which is robust in adults (human or otherwise), is inconsistent or absent in young children.

Keeping these cautions in mind, animal studies have been of great value in delineating the origins of evoked potentials. This chapter presents studies that used a variety of approaches to elucidate the generators of these potentials. Here, as elsewhere in this book, excerpts of the original studies are summarized or used verbatim where appropriate, as indicated by the footnotes to the text. Details of methodology are generally omitted. References and figures have been renumbered for consistency.

Origin of Auditory Brainstem Responses

Although there have been many investigations on the generators of the ABR, ambiguities remain. In this study, we see the use of three techniques—near-field recording, ablation, labeling—applied to the problem.

Central Auditory Pathway Disorders. K. Kaga
doi: 978-4-431-26920-5_2, © Springer 2009

Table 1. Possible generators of ABR peaks in cats

Study	Year	P1	P2	P3	P4	P5
Jewett	1970	Ipsi. AN	Near CN	Near SO	In and on either side	IC
Buchwald et al.	1975	Ipsi. AN	Ipsi. CN	Contra. SO	Both ICs	Contra. IC
Achor and Starr	1980	Ipsi. AN	Ipsi. CN Ipsi. CN	SO trazepoid body		
Caird et al.	1985				SO	
Fullerton and Kiang	1990				LL	
Melcher and Kiang	1996	Spiral ganglion	Ipsi. CN	CN	Both medial SOs	LL, IC
Kaga, Shinoda, et al.	1997	Ipsi. AN	Ipsi. CN Ipsi. SO	Contra. SO	Contra. SO LL	IC

Ipsi., ipsilateral; Contra., contralateral; AN, auditory nerve; CN, cochlear nucleus; SO, superior olivary complex; IC, inferior colliculus; LL, lateral lemniscal nucleus

Introduction[1]

Although the brainstem differs structurally between humans and small mammals (1), animal experiments are valuable for investigating generators of ABRs. Possible generators of each ABR peak in cats have been identified (Table 1) (2–10).

We designed three experiments to identify the origins of five peaks of ABRs in cats. In particular, we focused on the inferior colliculus (IC) because wave V of the human ABR is important clinically and because it is speculated that its generator is located in the IC (11).

The aim of the first experiment was to map out the auditory pathways within the brainstem through analysis of auditory evoked responses to click stimulation and for comparison ABRs. The second approach involved lesion studies to investigate changes in ABR wave configuration upon aspiration of the ICs and midline transection of the entire brainstem to investigate a role of the IC in the ABR. The third experiment was designed to study localization of brainstem auditory neurons projecting to the IC monosynaptically and forming ABR peaks resulting from IC activity injected Horse Radish Peroxidase.

Experiment 1: Whole Brainstem Mapping

The whole brainstem distribution of the responses in a plane of the IC to clicks delivered to the left ear in a cat is presented as an example in Fig. 1. This map indicates that large potentials are distributed around and in the auditory brainstem

---

[1]This section of the chapter was excerpted from: Kaga K, Shinoda Y Suzuki J-I. Origin of auditory brainstem responses in cats: whole brainstem mapping, and a lesion and HRP study of the inferior colliculus. *Acta Otolaryngol (Stockh)* 117:197–201, 1997. By permission.

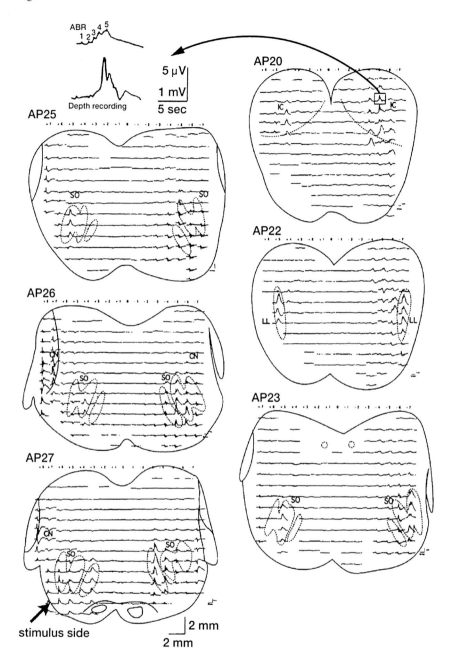

Fig. 1. Example of the distribution of field potentials at the level of the inferior colliculus (IC). *Arrow* indicates the stimulated ear. Large evoked potentials are recorded from auditory nuclei in the midbrain and brainstem. *SO*, superior olivary complex; *CN*, cochlear nucleus; *IC*, inferior colliculus; *LL*, lateral lemniscal nucleus

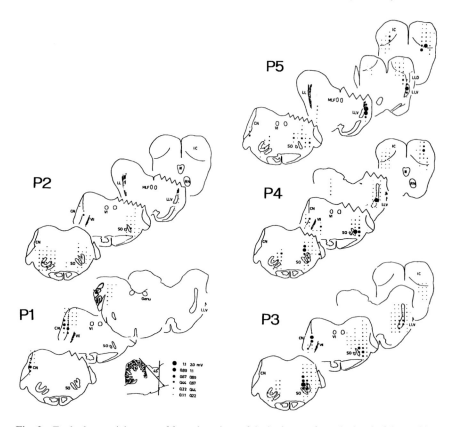

Fig. 2. Evoked potentials maps of frontal sections of the brainstem from the level of the cochlear nuclei to the level of the midbrain are constructed using whole brainstem field-potential analysis for comparison with auditory brainstem response (ABR) peaks. The diameter of each *dot* indicates the amplitude of the auditory evoked potentials, which correspond to each wave of ABRs at the corresponding site. Microvolt equivalents are given below. *VII*, facial nerve; *VI*, oculomotor nucleus; *LLV*, ventral lateral lemniscal nucleus; *LLD*, dorsal lateral lemniscal nucleus

necleus or tracts on the side contralateral to the stimulus side. The response is displayed more quantitatively in detail in Fig. 2, where the diameter of each dot indicates the amplitude of the auditory evoked potentials recorded in that plane and correspond to each ABR peak latency. The latency for the maximum amplitude of each auditory evoked potential varied from point to point in the auditory brainstem pathway. Therefore, the amplitude of each potential at each spot was defined as the amplitude at ABR peaks obtained anywhere over the scalp in that cat. The results were similar in other cats. They indicate that each ABR peak is comprised of evoked potentials originating from multiple auditory brainstem nuclei and tracts.

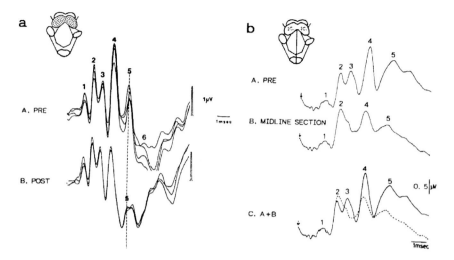

Fig. 3. a ABRs of a cat to monoaural stimulation before and after aspiration of both ICs. There is no effect up to and including P4, but the amplitude of P5 was markedly reduced after aspiration. **b** ABRs of a cat to monoaural stimulation before and after midline transactions of the brainstem and midbrain. P3 disappeared almost completely, and the amplitudes of P4 and P5 were reduced by up to one-half

Figure 3a shows the ABRs of one cat to monaural stimulation before and after aspiration of both ICs. There is no effect up to and including P4, but the amplitude of P5 is markedly reduced. Figure 3b shows that P3 disappeared almost completely, and the amplitudes of P4 and P5 were reduced by up to one-half.

Field-potential analysis to determine the site of phase reversal at which horseradish peroxidase (HRP) should be injected through a microsyringe was conducted in advance (Fig. 4). Common findings in six kittens were the following: 1) heavily HRP-labeled neurons were found in the contralateral lateral lemniscal nucleus, both superior olivary complexes (medial and lateral nucleus), and the cochlear nucleus ipsilateral to the stimulus side (Fig. 5); and 2) lightly HRP-labeled neurons were found in the ipsilateral IC and the contralateral cochlear nucleus (Fig. 5). (In all cases, ipsilateral and contralateral describe sites in regard to the stimulus side.)

Our data suggest that each peak wave consists of evoked potentials originating from multiple auditory brainstem nuclei and tracts. The potentials recorded in the present study are similar to those reported by other authors (4, 6, 8–11). However, whole brainstem mapping reveals that evoked potentials are elicited exclusively from auditory nuclei and tracts, and moreover, that each auditory nucleus elicits potentials, the latency range of which extends to multiple ABR peaks.

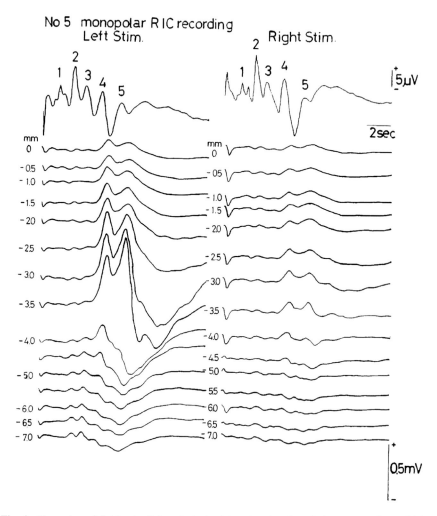

Fig. 4. Examples of field-potential analysis to determine the site of phase reversal at which horseradish peroxide (HRP) should be injected through a microsyringe

Experiment 2: IC Aspiration and Brainstem Midline Section

The results obtained in Experiment 2 after IC aspiration are similar to those obtained in previous studies; that is, IC aspiration had no effect on ABR waves up to and including P4 and resulted in reduced P5 amplitude (3, 6) (Fig. 3). The results after midline transection of the brainstem also revealed the disappearance of P3 and reduced amplitude of P4 and P5. These results suggest that generators of P5 are both ICs.

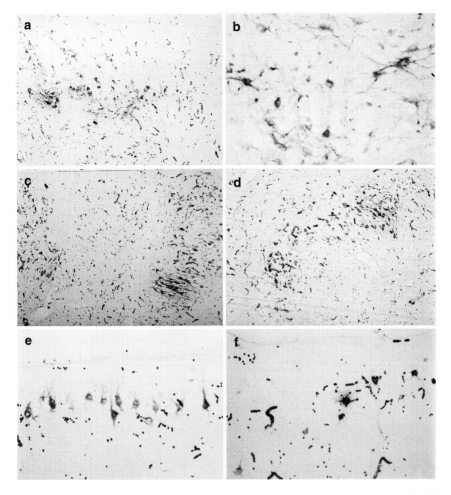

Fig. 5. a Lightly HRP-labeled cells are observed in the ipsilateral IC. **b–f** Heavily HRP-labeled cells in the brainstem auditory nuclei are observed in the lemniscal nucleus contralateral to the stimulus side (**b**); ipsilateral superior olivary complex (medial nucleus) (**c**); contralateral superior olivary complex (medial nucleus) (**d**); ipsilateral cochlear nucleus (**e**); and contralateral cochlear nucleus (**f**). "Contralateral" and "ipsilateral" refer to the stimulus side, not to the HRP injection site

Ten adult cats were used for this experiment. The entire method is the same as that for Experiment 1. Aspiration was performed to destroy both ICs of five cats. The brainstem was transected along the midline from the level of the IC to the cochlear nucleus and from dorsal to ventral using a specially made scalpel, and the ABRs were compared.

Experiment 3: HRP Injection to the Inferior Colliculus

In Experiment 3, analysis of field potentials in the IC showed that phase reversal of evoked potentials appeared in the central nucleus of the IC and the time of onset corresponds to P5 (Fig. 4). As revealed in this HRP study, P5, which was mainly elicited by electrical activity in the central nucleus of the IC, could be transduced by the summation of firings of monosynaptically innervated ascending neurons to the contralateral IC from the ipsilateral cochlear nucleus, both olivary complexes, and the ipsilateral nucleus (contralateral and ipsilateral to the stimulus sides) (Fig. 5). Based on these findings it is speculated that P5 must be driven initially by activity ascending neurons from the ipsilateral cochlear nucleus and from the ipsilateral lemniscal nucleus and bilateral olivary complexes (Fig. 5).

Comments

Based on the data of these three experiments, the main generators of each wave are proposed as follows: P1—ipsilateral cochlear nerves and cochlear nucleus; P2—ipsilateral cochlear nucleus and superior olivary complex; P3—contralateral superior olivary complex; P4—contralateral olivary complex and lateral lemniscus nucleus; and P5—both ICs.

Finally, this study illustrates the complexity of the problem of assigning specific generators to individual waves of the ABR. Other investigators have taken an interesting approach to the problem of identifying the generators in humans. By recording the ABR with three orthogonal pairs of electrodes—in X, Y, and Z axes—it is possible to create a three-dimensional display that shows the equivalent generator for each wave. An "equivalent generator" need not have a specific anatomical counterpart, however. If a wave has two or more generators, the equivalent generator is a single hypothetical source that would yield the same results. Although this research has been useful for illustrating the approximate location of the pathways involved, it is not used clinically. The necessary software is not widely available; more importantly, excellent recording conditions are required to generate accurate three-dimensional images.

References

1. Moore JK (1987) The human auditory brain stem: a comparative view. Hear Res 29:1–32
2. Jewett DL (1970) Volume-conducted potentials in response to auditory stimuli as detected by averaging in the cat. Electroencephalogr Clin Neurophysiol 28:609–618
3. Buchwald JS, Huang CM (1975) Far-field acoustics response: origins in the cat. Science 189:382–384
4. Achor LJ, Starr A (1980) Auditory brain stem responses in the cat. I. Intracranial and extra-cranial recordings. Electroencephalogr Clin Nuerophysiol 48:174–190
5. Achor LJ, Starr A (1980) Auditory brain stem responses in the cat. II. Effects of lesions. Electroencephalogr Clin Neurophysiol 48:174–190
6. Caird D, Sontheimer D, Klinke R (1985) Intra- and extracranially recorded auditory evoked potentials in the cat. I. Source location and binaural interaction. Electroencephalogr Clin Neurophyusiol 61:50–60
7. Fullerton BF, Kiang NYS (1990) The effect of brain stem lesions on brain stem auditory evoked potentials in the cat. Hear Res 49:363–390
8. Melcher JR, Knudson IM, Fullerton BC, et al (1996) Generators of the brain stem auditory evoked potential in cat. I. An experimental approach to their identification. Hear Res 93:1–27
9. Melcher JR, Guinan JJ Jr, Knudson IM, et al (1996) Generators of the brain stem auditory evoked potential in cat. II. Correlating lesion sites with waveform change. Hear Res 93:28–51
10. Melcher JR, Kiang NYS (1996) Generators of the brain stem auditory evoked potential in cat. III. Identified cell populations. Hear Res 93:52–71
11. Starr A, Hamilton AE (1976) Correlation between confirmed sites of neurological lesions and abnormalities of far-field auditory brain stem responses. Electroencephalogr Clin Neuro-physiol 41:595–608

Origin of Middle Latency Response

The middle latency response (MLR) exemplifies the ambiguities sometimes seen with evoked potentials: maturational effects in humans, multiple generators (one or more of which is affected by the sleep state), and questions as to whether the generators in humans are the same as in laboratory animals.

Middle latency responses are vertex-recorded auditory evoked responses (AEPs) detectable at 9–10 to 50–80 ms in humans (1–4). The origin of the MLR has been the source of continuing debate, and the development of a clinical testing technique has been seriously hampered. In patients with unilateral temporal lobe lesions involving the primary auditory cortex (AI), hemispheric asymmetry of the PA of the MLR has been described, and the bilateral temporal lobes are considered to be the source of the PA (5, 6). In some patients with bilateral lesions of the AI, the PA wave after Na wave of the MLR has been shown to be abolished (7–9). In contrast,

---

²This section of the chapter was excerpted from: Kim LS, Kaga K, Tsuzuku T, Uno A (1993) Effects of primary auditory cortex lesions on middle latency responses in awake cat. *Auris Nasus Larynx* 20:155–165.

in other potentials also with bilateral lesions, the PA has remained intact (10–12). In studies of animal lesions, Kaga et al. (13) showed that the cat PA is generated by the AI contralateral to the stimulated ear in the chloralose/urethane-anesthetized cat. On the other hand, Buchwald (14) showed that the AI is the generator of wave 7 in the awake cat. These conflicting results from human and animal studies raise questions about the role of the AI in the generation of MLRs. Comparisons among studies are also complicated by methodological differences, such as the recording site and the type of anesthesia employed.

Experiment

The aim of the present study was to clarify the role of the AI in MLRs. For this purpose we recorded auditory evoked potentials (AEPs) from the vertex of the skull on the right and left AI areas at various sites before and after creating serial lesions of the contralateral and ipsilateral AIs in awake cats.

To clarify the role of the primary AI on MLRs, we recorded the AEPs from the vertex and the right and left AI areas of the skull simultaneously before and after creating serial lesions of the AIs contralateral and ipsilateral to the stimulated ear in seven awake cats. The ABRs and MLRs recorded from the vertex in normal awake cats revealed the presence of peaks 1–8, NA wave, and PA wave during the analysis time of 50 ms (Fig. 1). After there were serial AI lesions: 1) all the peaks remained at nearly the same latencies; 2) the amplitude of the NA was decreased significantly, that of the PA was slightly decreased, and those of peaks 6, 7, and 8 were variable; and 3) the difference between the effects of the first operation

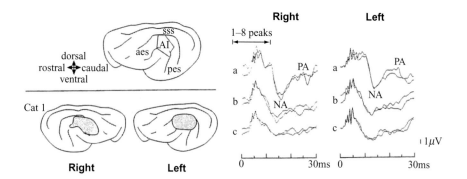

Fig. 1. Cat auditory brainstem responses (ABRs) and middle latency responses (MLRs) recorded from the vertex electrode, contralateral AI electrode, and ipsilateral AI electrode elicited by left click stimulation in an awake state and a Nembutal-anesthetized (*NA*) state. *sss*, suprasylvian sulcus; *aes*, anterior ectosylvian sulcus; *pes*, posterior ectosylvian sulcus

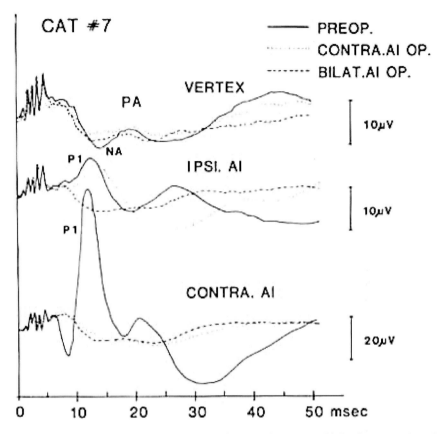

Fig. 2. Typical ABRs and MLRs of the preoperative (*PREOP.*) state and following a contralateral AI lesion (*CONTRA. AI OP.*) and bilateral AI lesions (*BILAT. AI OP.*) in an awake cat. Note that all the peaks are present after there is an AI lesion

(contralateral AI) and the second operation (ipsilateral AI) was not statistically significant (Fig. 2). These findings indicated that the main, prominent effect of bilateral AI lesions on MLRs in the awake cat is a significant decrease in the NA amplitude.

Comment

Our data showed that after the formation of bilateral AI lesions in awake cats all the peaks remained at nearly the same latencies, the amplitude of NA decreased significantly, the amplitude of PA decreased slightly, and the amplitudes of peaks

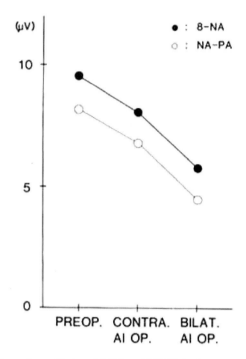

Fig. 3. Mean peak-to-peak amplitudes of 8-NA and NA-PA in the preoperative (*PREOP.*) state and after a contralateral AI lesion (*CONTRA. AI OP.*) in awake cats

6, 7, and 8 were variable (Fig. 3). These findings suggest that direct activation of the contralateral and ipsilateral AI in the awake cat results in large positive waves—P1s at 12–15 ms—in AI recordings, which were volume-conducted to the vertex as the NA following peak 8. In this study, the auditory evoked potentials recorded from he AI electrodes showed peaks 1–6 of ABRs and a small negative deflection around 8–9 ms followed by a large surface positive peak. P1 was at 12–15 ms, which is thought to be locally generated, as previous studies have described (14).

The PA wave in humans shows latency, a recovery cycle, and state-dependent properties (3) that are similar to those of wave "A" in the cat (14). Abnormalities in human Pa wave of MLRs are associated with subcortical lesions, not necessarily with the primary auditory cortex (12), whereas our present study showed that the AI is not the main generator of the PA in cats. The amplitude of a human PA is known to be significantly decreased in the presence of general anesthesia with halothane and enflurane, and the cat PA was observed to disappear during general anesthesia with Nembutal, as seen in Fig. 1. The data suggest that human PA could be analogous to cat PA wave and monkey Pa wave (Fig. 4) (15). Our results, together with those mentioned above, suggest that the primary auditory cortex in humans could be the generator of P_0, NA, and/or PA of the human MLR.

Over the years, attempts have been made to use the MLR clinically as a hearing test for infants and young children. These efforts have proven futile because the

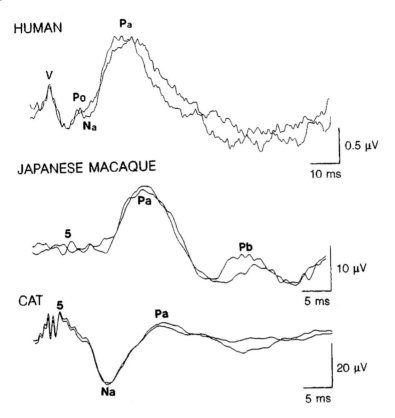

Fig. 4. Typical MLRs in awake humans, the Japanese macaque, and the cat. In the cat and Japanese macaque, responses were recorded from an electrode implanted on the skull on the vertex. Other recording conditions for the cat were the same as those for the monkey. Responses in the human were recorded from a silver cup electrode placed on the head skin of the vertex. Responses were averaged 500 times and analyzed within 100 ms[15]

generator that is so robust in adults is absent in young children. The remaining potential is labile, disappearing during certain sleep states; and it is virtually essential that the infant be asleep during the test to avoid myogenic artifacts. In neurological applications, clinicians have erred by assuming that the absence of the MLR in infants reflected a central nervous system abnormality.

References

1. Geisler CD, Frishkof LS, Rosenblith WA (1958) Extracranial responses to acoustic clicks in man. Science 128:1210–1211
2. Goldstein R, Rodman L (1967) Early components of averaged evoked responses to rapidly repeated auditory stimuli. J Speech Hear Res 10:697–705

3. Picton TW, Hillyard SA, Krausz HI, et al (1974) Human auditory evoked potentials. I. Evaluation of components. Elecroencephalogr Clin Neurophysiol 36:178–190
4. Özdamar O, Kraus N (1983) Auditory middle-latency responses in human. Audiology 22:34–49
5. Kraus N, Özdamar O, Hier D, et al (1982) Auditory middle latency responses (MLRs) in patients with cortical lesions. Electroencephalogr Clin Neurophysiol 54:275–287
6. Kile P, Paccioretti D, Wilson AF (1987) Effects of cortical lesions on middle-latency auditory evoked responses (MLRs). Elecroencephalogr Clin Neurophysiol 66:108–120
7. Graham J, Greenwood R, Lecky B (1980) Cortical deafness: a case report and review of he literature. J Neurol Sci 48:35–49
8. Shindo M, Kaa K, Tanaka Y (1981) Auditory agnosia following bilateral temporal lobe lesions: report of a case (in Japanese with English abstract). No to Shinkei 33:139–147
9. Özdamar O, Karuas N, Curry F (1982) Auditory brain seem and middle latency responses in a patient with cortical deafness. Electroencephalogr Clin Neurophysiol 53:224–230
10. Parving A, Salomon G, Elberling C, et al (1980) Middle components of he auditory evoked responses in bilateral temporal lobe lesions. Scand Audiol 9:161–167
11. Woods DL, Knight RT, Neville HJ (1984) Bitemporal lesions dissociate auditory evoked potentials and perception. Electroencephalogr Clin Neurophysiol 57:208–220
12. Woods DL, Clayaworth CC, Knight RT, et al (1987) Generators of middle- and long-latency auditory evoked potentials: implications from studies of patients with bitemporal lesions. Electroencephalogr Clin Neurophysiol 68:132–148
13. Kaga K, Hink RD, Shinoda Y, et al (1980) Evidence of a primary cortical origin of middle-latency auditory evoked potentials in cats. Elecroencephalogr Clin Neurophysiol 50:254–266
14. Buchwald JS (1983) Auditory evoked responses in clinical populations and in the cat. Auris Nasus Larynx (Tokyo) 10:87–95
15. Uno A, Kaga K, Tsuzuku T, et al (1993) Middle-latency responses of awake and anesthetized Japanese macaques. Audiology 32:302–307

3
Development and Brainstem Responses (ABRs)

By far, the most common clinical applications of evoked responses have been the use of the auditory brainstem response (ABR) to assess hearing in infants and young children.

Development of the Auditory Brainstem Response[1]

We begin with studies addressing pediatric audiological aspects. The cochlea is essentially mature long before birth, and ABRs can be recorded consistently after 32 weeks of gestation. However, the ABRs, or more precisely the underlying neural pathways, continue to mature for many months. An appreciation of the normal maturational process is necessary to interpret the ABR properly. Although many investigators have examined maturational effects on the latencies of the response with high stimulus levels, there is little information on the changes in ABR threshold during the first months of life. In addition to measuring the ABR threshold, this study also reports behavioral thresholds. Note how high the behavioral thresholds are despite normal cochlear function.

In a study of human brainstem evoked potentials, Hecox and Galambos (1) reported a progressive decline in the latency of wave V from 3 weeks to around 2 years of age. Salamy et al. (2, 3) compared brainstem evoked potentials among newborns, young infants, and adults. They also observed shortening of the peak latency (waves I and V) from birth to adulthood. Moreover, they demonstrated that the early and late components mature at different rates. These studies, however, failed to report how these ABR changes relate to behavioral development. This issue is of prime importance clinically, where behavioral methods of measuring hearing in infants have rather low reliability because of neurological or psychological factors (4).

---

[1]Much of this section of the chapter was excerpted from Kaga K, Tanaka Y. Auditory brainstem response and behavioral audiometry: developmental correlates. *Arch Otolaryngol* 106:564–566, 1980. By permission.

Central Auditory Pathway Disorders. K. Kaga
doi: 978-4-431-26920-5_3, © Springer 2009

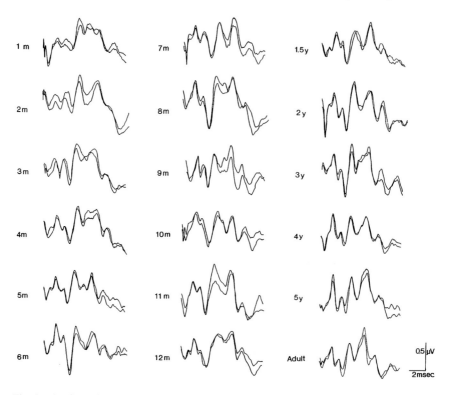

Fig. 1. Configuration changes in the auditory brainstem response (ABR) at the 85-dB hearing level. Each trace represents a typical response for the age indicated

The purpose of this study was to investigate the influence of human development on the ABR threshold and behavioral sensitivity changes from the first year of life to adulthood. The results should prove helpful in elucidating the relation between the development of the ABR and that of auditory behavior.

Developmental correlates of ABRs and behavioral audiometry in 112 normal subjects consisting of 78 infants (ages 1–18 months), 24 children (ages 2–5 years), and 10 adults (ages 18–22 years) were studied to provide normative data for audiological and neurological applications (Fig. 1). Thresholds of ABR, as determined by minimum stimulus intensities evoking wave V, decreased with age. Neonates had the highest ABR thresholds, and adults had the lowest (Fig. 2). The pattern for behavioral sensitivity was similar to that for ABR thresholds. Response functions determined by both methods converged with age. They crossed between the ages of 2 and 3 years. There was a trend for all peak latencies to decrease with age (Fig. 3), an effect that was particularly pronounced for the later ABR components.

Thresholds of ABR, as determined by minimum intensities evoking wave V, decreased with age. Neonates had the highest thresholds, and adults had the lowest. By the age of 2–3 years, the thresholds were comparable to those of adults. The

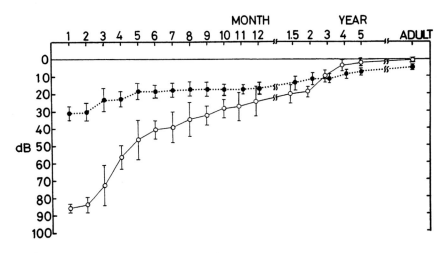

Fig. 2. Changes in the mean ABR thresholds for click and behavioral responses for 1- and 2-kHz pure tones with age. *Dotted line* shows ABR thresholds; *solid line* reflects behavioral sensitivity

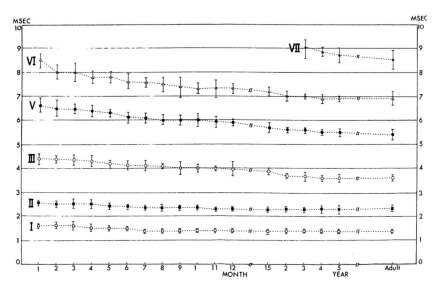

Fig. 3. Peak latency changes of waves I, II, III, V, and VI at the 85-dB hearing level as a function of age

cause of this decrease in wave V threshold may be progressive myelination, which results in a greater degree of synchronization among impulses arriving at the wave V generators. This interpretation is supported by the result that peak latencies decreased with age. Such a finding would be predicted by augmentation of nerve conduction velocity through myelination. Hecox and Galambos (1) suggested that increases in dendritic arborization and fiber diameter growth might also underlie the developmental changes of the ABR. Both of these factors could enhance synchronization, as does myelination, by reducing the conduction time. However, myelination does seem to be of prime importance because demyelinating diseases (5, 6) can reverse, to a large extent, the changes associated with development.

One can appreciate the impact that the ABR has made on pediatric audiology. Imagine the impossibility of assessing auditory function on the basis of behavioral thresholds. Could a correction factor be used if we know that the behavioral threshold is elevated by, for example, 40 dB at 6 months of age? No. With sensory loss, recruitment is seen—the rapid growth of loudness at suprathreshold intensities. An infant with a 60-dB loss might respond at 65 dB. Subtracting the 40-dB "correction factor" from 65 dB would greatly underestimate the impairment.

References

1. Hecox K, Galambos R (1974) Brainstem auditory evoked responses in human infants. Arch Otolaryngol 99:30–33
2. Salamy A, McKean DM, Buda FB (1975) Maturational changes in auditory transmission as reflected in human brain stem potentials. Brain Res 96:361–366
3. Salamy A, McKean CM (1976) Postnatal development of human brain stem potentials during the first year of life. Electroencephalogr Clin Neurophysiol 40:418–426
4. Hodgson WR (1978) Testing infants and young children. In: Katz J (ed) Handbook of clinical audiology. Williams & Wilkins, Baltimore, pp 397–409
5. Stockard MM, Rossiter VS (1977) Clinical and pathological correlates of brain stem auditory response abnormalities. Neurology 27:315–325
6. Kaga K, Tokoro Y, Tanaka Y, et al (1980) The progress of adrenoleucodystrophy as revealed by auditory evoked responses and brainstem histology. Arch Otorhinolaryngol 228:17–27

ABR in Preterm Infants[2]

Preterm infants are often at risk for hearing impairment. They may experience hypoxia, hyperbilirubinemia, or intraventricular hemorrhage. Life-saving antibiotics and certain other drugs may be ototoxic. Many of these risk factors have the potential to affect neural generators of the ABR as well as receptor cells. The norms for ABR latency in preterm infants have been published by others. Here we ask whether hearing and the ABR mature normally in preterm infants who have been spared insults to the cochlea and brainstem.

Auditory brainstem responses and behavioral thresholds were studied in 25 preterm infants at postconceptional ages of approximately 40 weeks to ascertain if

[2]Much of this section of the chapter was exerpted from Kaga K, Hashira S, Marsh RR. Auditory brainstem responses and behavioural responses in pre-term infants. *Br J Audiol* 20:121–127, 1986.

there were differences in the ABR between normal preterm and full-term newborns. The aim was to compare behavioral thresholds at around 40 weeks' postconceptional age and to follow changes in their behavioral thresholds during the first year of life. ABR thresholds, peak latencies of waves I and V, and the I–V peak interwave latency were measured. Behavioral audiometric thresholds to pure tones were determined through behavioral observation audiometry and conditioned orientation-reflex audiometry. The ABR thresholds of the preterm infants, whether they were small-for-dates (SFD) or appropriate-for-dates (AFD), were in the normal ranges of the controls (Fig. 1). Moreover, there were no significant differences between either the SFD group or the AFD group and the controls in terms of the wave I or V latency or the I–V interval (Figs. 2, 3). Thus, the ABR was apparently unaffected by the infant being SFD (Table 1).

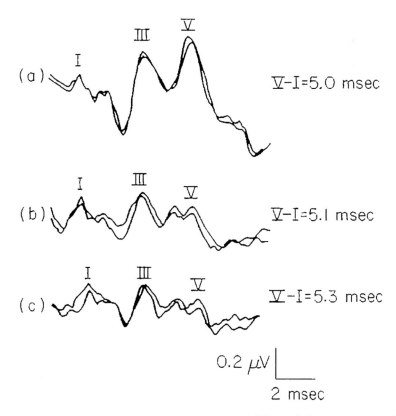

Fig. 1. Auditory brainstem responses (ABRs) of a normal full-term infant (**a**), an appropriate-for-dates (AFD) infant (**b**), and a small-for-dates (SFD) infant (**c**). Note that there was almost no difference in the peak intervals for wave I–V. **a** Full-term infant: birth weight 3200 g; postnatal age 6 days; postconceptional age 40 weeks. **b** ASFD infant: birth weight 1720 g; postnatal age 4 weeks; postconceptional age 33 weeks. **c** SFD infant: birth weight 1894 g; postnatal age 2 weeks; postconceptional age 39 weeks

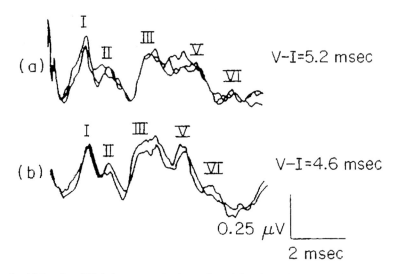

Fig. 2. ABRs of an AFD infant at ages (**a**) 2 months and (**b**) 12 months. Birth weight was 1020 g, and the gestational period was 28 weeks

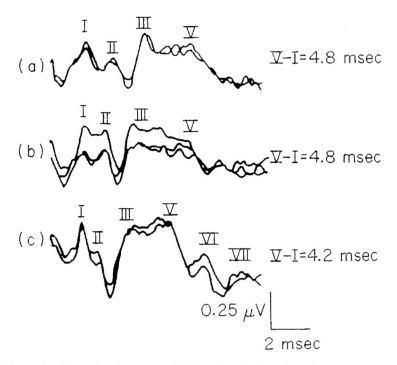

Fig. 3. ABRs of an SFD infant at ages (**a**) 2 months, (**b**) 5 months, and (**c**) 12 months. Birth weight was 1400 g, and the gestational period was 35 weeks

Behavioral audiometry disclosed that all normal full-term infants responded to pure-tone stimuli, with mean thresholds of 85 dB, whereas only 42% of AFD infants and 30% of SFD infants responded to pure-tone stimuli at ≤90 dB (Fig. 4). With the exception of a few infants, behavioral thresholds caught up with the normal range by 12 months of age.

The gestational age and birth weight of premature infants varies, but the peak latencies and the central conduction time (wave I–V peak interval) are more prolonged with the earlier gestational age at birth (1). However, our cross-sectional data showed no difference between ABR maturation inside and outside the uterus so long as the ABRs of preterm and full-term newborns are compared at around ≥40 weeks' gestational age (2). In addition, the ABR was apparently unaffected by

Table 1. Mean gestational age at birth and postconceptional age at the time of ABR examinations

Infant group	No.	Gestational age at birth (weeks)	Postconceptional age at birth (weeks)
Normal: full term	6	41.0 ± 1.6	41.5 ± 2.0
Premature			
Appropriate for dates	12	31.4 ± 3.0	39.3 ± 2.5
Small for dates	13	36.7 ± 1.8	41.6 ± 1.9

Results are given as the mean ± SD
ABR, auditory brainstem response

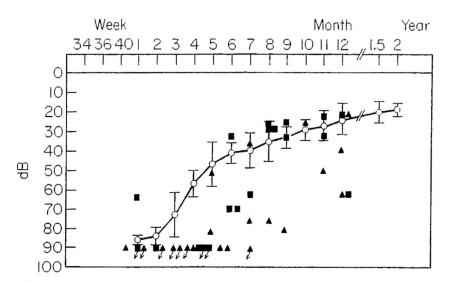

Fig. 4. Overall behavioral audiometry thresholds of 25 premature AFD (*solid triangles*) and SFD (*solid squares*) babies during the first year of the life, plotted with those of normal infants and adults (*open circles* and *solid lines*)

the infant being SFD, as Fawer and Dobowitz (3) reported. These findings suggest that maturation of the ABR is highly dependent on the postconceptional age, rather than the age at birth or the postnatal weight.

The electroencephalographic (EEG) response to clicks during sleep was reported in a group of normal premature infants in a longitudinal study. The decreasing latency of the responses and changes in waveform characteristics as the infants mature permit reliable estimation of the postconceptional age during approximately 4-week periods (4). Therefore, both brain maturation evaluated by EEG and brain-stem maturation evaluated by ABR can be correlated with the postconceptional age of the infants.

On the other hand, our cross-sectional and follow-up data showed great differences in the thresholds determined by behavioral audiometry. At around 40 weeks, all normal full-term babies responded to pure-tone stimuli at 85 dB, but only 42% of AFD and 30% of SFD infants responded to pure tone-stimuli at ≤90 dB; the others showed no responses to pure-tone stimuli at 90 dB.

Preterm infants are not just at risk for hearing impairment; there may be other deficits as well, including developmental delay. ABR tests and knowledge of auditory development in this population can aid the neurologist or developmental pediatrician in assessing the child's neurological and developmental status (5).

References

1. Schulman-Galambos C Galambos R (1975) Brainstem auditory evoked responses in premature infants. J Speech Hearing Res 18:456–465
2. Starr A, Amlie RN, Martin WH, et al (1977) Development of auditory function in newborn infants revealed by auditory brainstem potentials. Pediatrics 60:813–839
3. Fawer C-L, Dobowitz LMS (1982) Auditory brainstem response in neurologically normal pre-term and full-term newborn infants. Neuropediatrics 13:200–206
4. Weizman ED, Grazinani L, Klig V, et al (1967) Spatiotemporal mapping of sensory evoked responses from the scalp EEG of premature infants. Neurology 17:310–318
5. Yakovlev PI, Lecours AR (1967) The myelogenetic cycles of regional maturation of the brain. In: Minkoweski A (ed) Regional development of the brain in early life. Blackwell, Oxford, pp 3–70

Progressive Hearing Impairment During Infancy

For reasons that are not well understood, some preterm infants develop hearing loss long after their discharge from the hospital. Here are two reports.

First Report[3]

Four high-risk infants who had normal ABRs at the time of discharge from the neonatal intensive care unit (NICU) were found at follow-up 18–23 months later to have significant hearing loss. Birth weights ranged from 2422 to 3220 g and gestational ages from 35 to 41 weeks. All of the infants required mechanical ventilation with severe respiratory difficulty. Three of the four had persistent pulmonary hypertension of the newborn (PPHN). Two infants were given aminoglycoside, three pancuronium bromide, and four furosemide. We concluded that infants who had severe respiratory difficulty may remain at risk for development of significant hearing loss even though they have passed an initial ABR screening test during the newborn period.

Congenital diaphragmatic hernia may cause progressive deafness (1, 2). In this study, three patients were studied until the end of preschool: two children wore hearing aids only, and one child underwent cochlear implant surgery (Table 1). Their hearing, speech, and language were evaluated by neuropsychological tests, which showed that hearing, speech, and language abilities were better in the child with the cochlear implant than in the two children with hearing aids (Table 2). Cochlear implants are thus recommended to improve hearing and speech in children with a congenital diaphragmatic hernia who develop progressive deafness after surgery.

Table 1 Pre-school age education of a cochlear implant case

Parameter	Data
Diagnosis	Congenital diaphragmatic hernia
Birth weight	2564 g
Diagnosis	Profound hearing loss
ABR	
Two months old	R: 80 dB, L: 60 dB
Two years old	R and L, no responses
Hearing aid fitting	2 years 9 months
Preschool education	Auditory oral
PTA	R: 116 dB, L: 120 dB
Cochlear implant	3 years 11 months
Preschool education	Special school for hearing-impaired children
Communication	Auditory oral

R, right; L, left; ABR, auditory brainstem response; PTA, pure tone average

[3]This section of the chapter was excerpted from Shinjou Y, Kaga K. Four cases of progressive hearing loss after discharge from NICU. *Otol Jpn* 12:212–216. By permission.

Table 2. Neuropsychological examination of a cochlear implant case

Verbal IQ vs. performance IQ	
At 3 years 11 months of age (1 year after auditory oral training)	
K Development Test	
Cognitive age: 3 years and 9 months	
Performance developmental quotient: 88	
Verbal age: 1 year and 9 months	
Verbal developmental quotient: 44	
At 6 years of age	
WPPSI Test	
Performance IQ:	106
Verbal IQ:	55
At 8 years of age	
WISC-R test	
Performance IQ:	118
Verbal IQ:	72
Auditory perception at present	
Monosyllables	65%
Words	92%
Sentences	94%
Environmental sounds	75%

IQ, intelligence quotient; WPPSI, Wechsler Preschool and Primary Scale of Intelligence; WISC-R, Wechsler Intelligence Scale for Children—Revised

Second Report[4]

We herein report the case of a 14-month-old infant who was diagnosed as having progressive hearing loss by repeatedly assessing his ABRs during his 1-year stay in the NICU. He was born prematurely with asphyxia, hyperbilirubinemia, and respiratory distress. During his year in the NICU he was under constant mechanical ventilation. Repeated ABRs over this year initially showed normal waves but subsequently demonstrated progressive hearing impairment, leading finally to no responses (Fig. 1). Possible causes of this progressive deafness include the multiple problems of asphyxia, hyperbilirubinemia, and pulmonary disorder.

Comments

ABRs have revealed newly various diseases with progressive hearing impairments in infancy. These two case reports describe only typical diseases among many.

---

[4]This section of the chapter was excerpted from Huang L, Kaga K, Hashimoto K. Progressive hearing loss in an infant in a neonatal intensive care unit as revealed by auditory evoked brainstem responses. *Auris Nasus Larynx* 29:187–190.

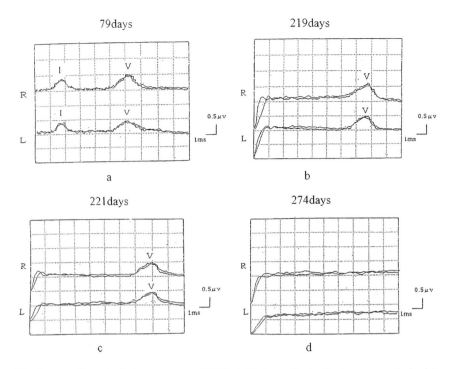

Fig. 1. **a** Auditory brainstem response (ABR) at 79 days after birth shows normal absolute latencies of waves I and V and a normal waves I–V interval, taking the infant's age into consideration. **b** ABR at 219 days after birth indicates the loss of wave I and prolonged latency of wave V. **c** ABR at 221 days after birth illustrates continuing prolongation of wave V latency. **d** ABR at 274 days shows no response

References

1. Kawashiro N, Tsuchihashi N, Koga K, et al (1996) Delayed post-neonate intensive care unit hearing disturbance. Int J Otorhinolaryngol 34:35–43
2. Cheung PY, Tyebkhan JM, Peliowski A (1999) Prolonged use of pancuronium bromide and sensorineural hearing loss in childhood survivors of congenial diaphragmatic hernia. J Pediatr 135:233–239

4
Auditory Nerve Lesions

The auditory nerve is composed of the cochlear nerve and vestibular nerve, which run, respectively, from the cochlea to the cochlear nucleus and from the vestibular organs to the vestibular nucleus in the medulla oblongata. Because the auditory nerve is confined to the internal auditory canal (IAC) for part of its course, tumors in the IAC may damage the vestibular or cochlear branch no matter from which branch they originate. Unilateral acoustic neuromas are more common, but bilateral acoustic neurofibromas may be found in patients with neurofibromatosis type II.

Vestibular Schwannoma[1]

Electrocochleography (ECochG) and the auditory brainstem response (ABR) are electrophysiologically important tools in routine use for diagnosing vestibular schwannomas (1, 2). Results of studies of the temporal bone pathology of vestibular schwannoma have been reported from the viewpoint of histopathology (3–6) but rarely from the viewpoint of electrophysiology. ECochG and ABR, respectively, can provide important information on the origins of compound action potentials (CAPs) and wave I. We report a case of vestibular schwannoma in which ECochG and ABR were correlated with temporal bone pathology.

---

[1]This material was excerpted from: Kaga K, Iwasaki S, Tamura A, et al. Temporal bone pathology of acoustic neuroma correlating with presence of electrocochleography and absence of auditory brainstem response. *J Laryngol Otol* 111:967–972, 1997.

Case History

The temporal bone pathology of a 74-year-old woman affected by a vestibular schwannoma was compared with ECochG and ABR findings. At age 71, she complained of hearing loss in the left ear in which pure-tone audiometry revealed threshold elevation in the middle- and high-frequency range (Fig. 1). Temporal bone computed tomography (CT) revealed a medium-sized cerebellopontine angle tumor in the left ear (Fig. 2). ABR testing showed no response in the left ear, but ECochG showed clear compound action potentials (CAPs) (Fig. 3). Three years later, at age 74, she died of metastatic lung cancer and sepsis. The left temporal bone pathology consisted primarily of a large vestibular schwannoma occupying the internal auditory meatus (Fig. 4). The organ of Corti was well preserved in each cochlear turn (Fig. 5). In the modiolus, the number of spiral ganglion cells and cochlear nerve fibers were decreased in each cochlear turn.

These histological findings suggest that clear CAPs were recorded from the distal portion of the cochlear nerve despite the presence of the vestibular schwannoma, but ABRs could not be detected because of blockage of the proximal portion of the cochlear nerve by the vestibular schwannoma.

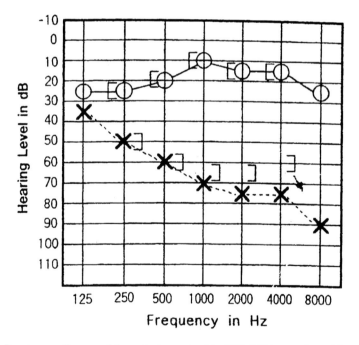

Fig. 1. Pure-tone audiogram of the patient examined in 1988. Mild sensorineural hearing loss with gradual threshold elevation in the high-frequency range was revealed for the left ear (*dotted line*), whereas the right ear exhibited normal hearing (*solid line*)

Fig. 2. Auditory brainstem response (*ABR*) and electrocochleography (*ECochG*). In the left ear, ABR at 100 dB hearing level (HL) elicited no response, but ECochG demonstrated clear compound action potentials at 100, 80, and 60 dB HL

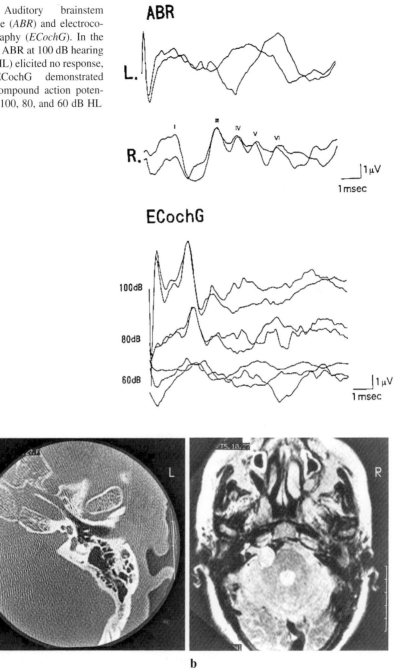

Fig. 3. Computed tomography (CT) (**a**) and magnetic resonance imaging (MRI) (**b**) demonstrated the presence of a medium-sized tumor in the left internal auditory canal and cerebellopontine angle

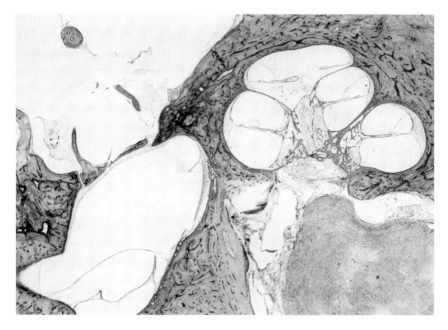

Fig. 4. Mid-modiolar section of the left ear revealed enlargement of the internal auditory canal, which was occupied by a vestibular schwannoma (*). (H&E, ×10)

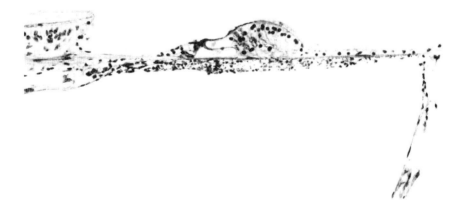

Fig. 5. Organ of Corti of the basal turn of the left cochlea shows that inner and outer hair cells are well preserved. (H&E, ×50)

Comment

In 1920, Antoni (cited in ref. 7) divided vestibular schwannomas into two histological types. Type A tumor is composed of merging and diverging streams of elongated
spindle cells, usually with large nuclei; there is a tendency for the nuclei to be
aligned in straight or curved rows with the long axes parallel to one another, resulting in a palisade pattern. Type B tumor is a degenerate form that is often inter-
mingled with type A tumor but can be well demarcated. It is characterized by a
loose texture and polymorphism of tumor cells. In our patient, the vestibular
schwannoma was classified as a mixture of type A and type B tumors because it
exhibited both a palisade pattern and loose texture.

Clinical and histological studies (6) indicate that there are at least three mechanisms responsible for auditory and vestibular dysfunction: 1) atrophy or destruction
of cochlear and vestibular nerve fibers due to the pressure of tumor invasion;
2) ischemia causing atrophy of the sense organs and labyrinth by compromising
blood flow in the labyrinthine artery; and 3) biochemical degradation of the fluids
of the inner ear as evidenced by the presence of an acidophilic substance in the
perilymphatic spaces on tissue preparations (7) and increased concentration of
protein substances in the perilymph (2). However, in the temporal bone of this
patient, destruction of vestibular and cochlear nerve fibers with the preservation
of vestibular end-organs and Corti's organ was observed. Moreover, the distal
portion of the cochlear nerve was demonstrated by ECochG to be functioning,
but the proximal portion was not, as shown by ABR testing. The reason that
wave I on the ABR test was not observed was because of the low amplitude of
the CAPs.

Shanon et al. (8) described a relation between tumor size and ECochG-demon-
strated CAP morphology. Small or medium-sized tumors left preserved CAPs, with
normal or sometimes enhanced amplitude. Cochlear microphonic activity was
present even with severe hearing loss, as assessed by pure-tone audiometry. For
large tumors, the CAP amplitude was diminished, and N1 of the CAP became broad
and less well defined. With continued tumor growth, the CAP could become unde-
tectable. Presumably, this sequence of events is related to progressive pressure and
edema of the VIII nerve, and eventually disruption of the VIII nerve and cochlear
blood supply, which desynchronizes the response.

In our patient, the tumor was a large type (by Shanon's classification), but the
CAP was present. In Shanon et al.'s study, no temporal bone pathology was
described, but CT was used to compare the tumor size with the CAP seen by
ECochG.

The combined ECochG/ABR approach is particularly well suited to assess auditory function in VIII nerve tumors (2). In many studies, the types of ABR abnormality are compared to differentiate cochlear versus VIII nerve lesions using CT
or magnetic resonance imaging (MRI). However, more histological correlation
studies are needed to demonstrate the origins of the CAP seen by ECochG and the
wave I in the ABR. Temporal bone pathology studies on vestibular schwannomas

correlating the audiometry, ECochG, and early wave of ABR results can provide clues for exploring the origins of ECochG and ABR findings.

The ABR configuration of patients with an acoustic neuroma may be classified as no response, wave I only, wave I and II only, or prolongation of wave V-I brainstem conduction time. The configuration may change with the growth of the acoustic tumor, during acoustic neuroma surgery, or after acoustic neuroma extirpation. Note the test findings in this case: absent ABR and present cochlear microphonic activity. Consider, as you read the next section, whether these findings might have led some to diagnose unilateral auditory neuropathy.

References

1. Selters W, Brackmann DE (1977) Acoustic tumor detection with brainstem electric response audiometry. Arch Otolaryngol 103:181–187
2. Eggermont JJ, Don M, Brackmann DE (1980) Electrocochleography and auditory brainstem electric responses in patients with pontine angle tumours. Ann Otol Rhinol Laryngol 89:1–19
3. Benitez JT, Lopez Rios G, Novoa V (1967) Bilateal acoustic neuroma: a human temporal bone report. Arch Otolaryngol 86:25–31
4. De Moura L (1967) Inner ear pathology in acoustic neurinoma. Arch Otolaryngol 85:125–133
5. Suga F, Lindsay JR (1976) Inner ear degeneration in acoustic neurinoma. Ann Otol Rhinol Laryngol 85:343–358
6. Schuknecht HF (1993) Pathology of the ear. 2nd edn. Lea & Febiger, Philadelphia, pp 461–468
7. Yllikoski J, Collan Y, Palva T, et al (1978) Cochlear nerve in neurilemomas: audiology and histopathology. Arch Otolaryngol Head Neck Surg 104:679–684
8. Shanon E, Gold A, Himmelfarb MS (1981) Auditory brainstem responses in cerebellopontine angle tumors. Laryngoscope 91:254–259

Auditory Nerve Disease (Auditory Neuropathy)

In contrast to the focal lesions caused by compression from a tumor, there can be diffuse damage. It is known that the number of cochlear nerves diminish in elderly people, although it is by no means clear how much this contributes to presbycusis. It has also long been known that hearing is affected in some patients with peripheral neuropathy.

A new concept of auditory neuropathy or auditory nerve disease as a distinct entity was proposed in 1996. The term "auditory nerve disease" was proposed in a report by Kaga et al. in 1996 (1), and "auditory neuropathy" was proposed by Starr et al. that same year (2). These two terms refer to the same auditory disorder. A typical presentation of this disease includes a mild to moderate threshold elevation in pure-tone audiometry, extremely poor speech discrimination, normal distortion-product otoacoustic emissions (DPOAEs), the presence of summating potentials (–SP) but the absence of CAPs by ECochG, and the absence of ABRs. Note that the electrophysiological tests themselves are not sufficient to diagnose auditory neuropathy. The patient's history and audiological findings are relevant. In the series of Starr et al. (2), the diagnosis was confirmed in many cases by finding neuropathy elsewhere in the peripheral nerves.

Diagnosis of Auditory Nerve Disease[2]

The three patients discussed here had preserved electrocorticography (ECoG) results and otoacoustic emissions (OAEs), but their ABRs were essentially abolished. Their histories, hearing test results—audiography, speech intelligibility scores, tympanometry, stapedius reflex, auditory evoked potentials, OAEs—and neurological and radiological findings (CT, MRI) are summarized in Table 1.

Audiometrically, all patients had a low-frequency loss with a rising slope pattern, the severity of which ranged from mild to moderate. Speech discrimination scores were markedly abnormal (poor) in all patients despite mild to moderate elevation of the pure-tone audiograms, suggesting retrocochlear pathology (Fig. 1). Standard measures of tympanic membrane mobility (tympanometry) revealed normal patterns in all patients. The stapedius reflex thresholds in all patients were offscale (absent). ABRs were essentially absent bilaterally in all patients; however, one patient (patient 3) had a small response at 1 ms in the left ear at 100 dB nHL. Click-evoked ECoGs in all patients showed large negative summating potentials and small CAPs (only in patient 1) at intensities of 70–100 dB nHL (Fig. 2).

Table 1. Four test results of auditory speech discrimination, recognition, and comprehension

Test	Patient 1 (%)	Patient 2 (%)	Patient 3 (%)
Maximum speed discrimination in speech audiometry			
Right	35	20	45
Left	45	25	35
Word recognition test (25 words)	92	88	60
Short sentence comprehension test (10 sentences)	98	98	40
Token test[a] (De Renzi & Vignolo)	98	96	95

[a] De Renzi, Vignolo LA. The token test: a sensitive test to detect receptive disturbances in aphasics. *Brain* 85:665–678, 1962.

---

[2]This section of the chapter was abstracted and excerpted from: Kaga K, Nakamura M, Shinogami M, et al. Auditory nerve disease of both ears revealed by auditory brainstem responses, electrocochleography and otoacoustic emissions. *Scand Audiol* 25:233–238, 1996.
Note: The orginal publication described two cases. Their findings are summarized here along with those of a third, similar case. The discussion that follows is quoted from the publication directly—hence the mention of only two cases.

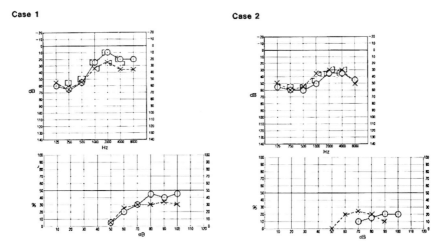

Fig. 1. Pure-tone and speech audiograms of patients 1 and 2. The speech audiogram is illustrated by a speech sound level on the horizontal axis and discrimination percentage for each decibel level on the vertical axis. There is a severe, disproportionate loss of intelligibility for speech

Transient evoked otoacoustic emissions (TEOAEs) and DPOAEs in patient 2 were normal (Fig. 3). In patient 1, left-ear TEOAEs were of low amplitude at 1, 2, and 6 kHz; DPOAEs were normal at 1–2 kHz, absent at 2–4 kHz, and of low amplitude at 4–6 kHz. In the right ear, TEOAEs were normal at 1–3 kHz, and DPOAEs were slightly reduced around 6 kHz. In patient 3, TEOAEs and DPOAEs were normal around 1–3 kHz bilaterally. No response was obtained from either ear at 3–8 kHz. The overall response amplitude was higher from the left ear. The results of our series of auditory and vestibular function tests suggest that in these patients lesions could exist at the auditory nerve but with slight involvement of the cochlear or vestibular organs and brainstem.

In general, most patients who show adult onset of combined auditory and vestibular damage of both ears are diagnosed as having suffered from the effects of ototoxic drugs, meningitis, bilateral acoustic tumors, Menière's disease, Friedreich's ataxia, or autosomal-dominant inheritance of inner ear disease. Unlike the background in such patients, no particular hereditary or pathological evidence was found in our patients; and even though the auditory-vestibular damage was longstanding and constant, it showed some subjective progression as they grew older. Although the pathology of the auditory-vestibular nerve damage in these patients is obscure, inner ear diseases of inherited and toxic disorders and Menière's disease can be almost ruled out. The main lesion could have been located in the auditory nerve or the synapses to hair cells, as ECochG demonstrated obvious negative summating potentials of broad type, with poor CAPs; ABRs of each ear to loud click were absent despite normal OAEs and almost normal DPOAEs.

At present, TEOAE and DPOAE are useful tools for evaluating the functioning of outer hair cells in middle- and high-frequency regions (≥1 kHz). Spectrum

Fig. 2. Auditory brainstem responses (ABRs) and electrocochleograms (EcochGs) of patients 1 and 2. ABRs are absent bilaterally in both patients. Regarding the EcochGs, both cases show negative summating potentials and small compound action potentials

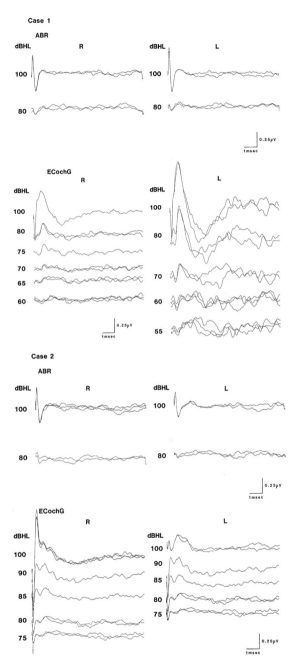

analysis of TEOAEs has shown significant correlations between the 1-kHz hearing level and spectrum components of the bands around 1 kHz (3). If a TEOAE is present in the frequency spectrum, the hearing level at 1 kHz is ≤35 dB (4). DPOAEs elicited by two primary tones, f1 and f2, were previously found to

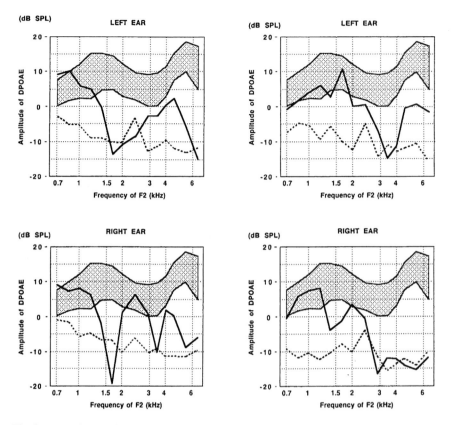

Fig. 3. Distortion-product otoacoustic emissions (DPOAEs) in patients 1 and 2 are shown by *solid lines*. Amplitudes of DPOAEs are within the normal range—around 1 kHz in all ears. Responses around 2 kHz are reduced in the left ear of patient 1 and are nearly normal in the right ear of patient 1 and both ears of patient 2. Responses around 4 kHz are reduced in both patients. The *dotted area* represents the mean ± SD of DPOAEs from 40 normal ears

correlate with the auditory threshold, or f2, frequency (5, 6). The low amplitudes of DPOAEs in the high-frequency region in patients 1 and 2 reflect outer hair cell dysfunction in the area. These mild sensory hearing losses in the high-frequency area are probably due to presbycusis. The amplitudes of DPOAEs and TEOAEs were more robust than expected from the corresponding hearing losses at 1 kHz in the left ear of patient 1 and at 1 and 2 kHz in that patient's right ear as well as in both ears of patient 2. The dissociation of hearing levels with corresponding OAEs in the middle-frequency area shows that the function of outer hair cells in the regions was normal; and it supports the presence of retrocochlear hearing loss at least in the middle-frequency area.

Comment

Schuknecht and Woellner (7) first showed that partial lesions of the feline cochlear nerve may be associated with normal hearing thresholds for pure tones. Subsequently, Jerger et al., including Schuknecht, suggested that this may also be true in humans (8, 9). They offered findings in subjects with VIII nerve tumors in whom the hearing thresholds for pure tones, although not normal, were not seriously affected. By contrast, however, there was a severe, disproportionate loss of intelligibility for speech. The authors attributed this deficit to cochlear nerve fiber degeneration, which normally results from these tumors accompanied by good preservation of the cells in Corti's organ. Citrom et al. (10) described comparable findings and suggested that although at normal threshold levels a full complement of normal hair cells is needed to initiate the cochlear action potentials only a few nerve fibers are needed to propagate them and thus subserve normal sensation. These previous studies suggest that our patients could have similar findings between the hearing thresholds for pure tones and a severe, disproportionate loss of intelligibility for speech. Thus, we propose that the tentative diagnostic term "auditory nerve disease" be used to describe this entity.

Since the reports of Kaga et al. (1) and Starr et al. (2), there has been considerable interest in auditory neuropathy in the audiology community, in part because it can now be detected by a combination of findings. The presence of OAEs or cochlear microphonic activity demonstrates the integrity of at least the outer hair cells of the cochlea, whereas absence of the ABR shows failure of the cochlea to generate a normal neural response. Unfortunately, this enthusiasm has led many to apply the diagnosis of AN in cases of inner hair cell dysfunction or even agenesis of the auditory nerve merely because the ABR and OAEs findings are similar to those in AN.

The distinction between inner hair cell impairment and auditory nerve disorder is quite important because the cochlear implant stimulates the cochlear nerve. Patients with inner hair cell dysfunction (e.g., due to a mutation of the otoferlin gene) can be expected to have excellent auditory nerve survival and good outcomes with cochlear implantation. The story is far less clear for true neuropathies. The literature on cochlear implantation in patients with AN is difficult to interpret because many of the "AN" cases may actually be cases of inner hair cell dysfunction.

Progress is being made in the differential diagnosis of auditory neuropathy from inner hair cell impairment. The history is important, as many neuropathies (e.g., Charcot-Marie-Tooth disease, Friedreich's ataxia) develop late in childhood or during adulthood. The inner hair cell disorders are congenital and seem to result in severe or profound hearing impairment. We can expect genetic and electrophysiological tests to confirm the diagnosis; already there are suggestions that ECochG might identify inner hair cell impairment. For one group of patients, however, the diagnosis remains ambiguous. Certain infants who had difficult perinatal courses (e.g., hyperbilirubinemia, respiratory distress) may have signs of auditory neuropathy, but it is still not known if the lesion is at the level of the inner hair cells, the auditory nerve, or both. There might also be lesions of the cochlear nucleus and other central nervous system insults as well.

References

1. Kaga K, Nakamura M, Shinogami M, et al (1996) Auditory nerve disease of both ears revealed by auditory brainstem responses, electrocochleography and otoacoustic emissions. Scand Audiol 25:233–238
2. Starr A, Piction TW, Sininger Y, et al (1996) Auditory neuropathy. Brain 119:741–753
3. Collet K, Veuillet E, Chanal JM, et al (1991) Evoked otoacoustic emissions: correlates between spectrum analysis and audiogram. Audiology 30:164–172
4. Hurley RM, Musiek FE (1994) Effectiveness of transient-evoked otoacoustic emissions (TEOAEs) in predicting hearing level. J Am Acad Audiol 5:195–203
5. Martin GM, Ohlms LA, Flanklin DF, et al (1990) Distortion product emissions in humans. III. Influence of sensorineural hearing loss. Ann Otol Rhinol Laryngol 99:30–42
6. Whitefield ML, McCoy MJ, Lonsbury-Martin BL, et al (1955) Dependence of distortion-product otoacoustic emissions on primary levels in normal and impaired ears. I. Effects of decreasing L_2 below L_1. J Acoust Soc Am 97:2346–2358
7. Schuknecht H, Woellner R (1955) An experimental and clinical study of deafness from lesions of the cochlear nerve. J Laryngol Otol 69:75–97
8. Jerger S, Jerger J (1980) Intracranial tumors affecting the central auditory system and multiple sclerosis. In: Auditory disorders, a manual for clinical evaluations. Little, Brown, Boston, pp 79–93
9. Jerger J, Neely JD, Jeger S (1981) Speech audiometry, and auditory brain stem response in auditory brain stem tumors: importance of a multiple-test strategy. Ann NY Acad Sci 374:412–420
10. Citrom L, Dix MR, Hoallpike CS (1976) A recent clinico-pathological study of cochlear nerve degeneration resulting from tumor pressure and disseminated sclerosis with particular reference to the finding of normal threshold sensitivity for pure tones. Acta Otolaryngol (Stockh) 56:330–337

5
Brainstem and Midbrain Lesions

When viewing drawings of the brainstem auditory pathways, it is easy to imagine that the brainstem is merely a series of telegraph stations relaying messages to the cortex. However, a significant amount of processing occurs at the brainstem level, and lesions can affect higher functions even if not all pathways to the cortex have been severed. There is another aspect of brainstem anatomy. The brainstem is small, the size of a man's thumb, and all but the tiniest lesions can be expected to affect multiple tracts or nuclei. In this chapter, a range of insults—from the subtle to the fatal—are considered.

ABR Abnormality and Speech Perception in Brainstem Lesions

The auditory evoked potentials, although valuable tools, do not replace more traditional tests. In the next two selections, ABR testing is used in concert with speech testing to delineate the effect of brainstem lesions. The report on palatal myoclonus highlights the close proximity of the many brainstem structures to one another.

Patients with Brainstem Lesions[1]

The ABR, along with a variety of audiometric tests, have been applied to patients affected by brainstem lesions or auditory central processing disorders. Stephens

---

[1]This section of the chapter was excerpted from: Kaga K, Shindo M, Tanaka Y. Auditory brain stem responses and nonsense monosyllable perception test findings for patients with auditory nerve and brain stem lesions. *Laryngoscope* 96:1272–1278, 1986.

and Thornton (1) reported that unilateral abnormalities in low redundancy speech tests, prolonged auditory reaction times, and reduced loudness growth on the alternate binaural loudness-balance test were revealed to ipsilateral wave IV abnormalities or contralateral wave V abnormalities of the ABR. Jerger and Jerger (2, 3) reported that the combination of normal or near-normal pure-tone sensitivity associated with an abnormal ABR is a strong retrocochlear sign. Musiek and Geurkink (4) reported that both the ABR and central auditory test batteries were highly sensitive to brainstem lesions in this patient group as a whole, but the conventional speech discrimination test was not sensitive because none of the subjects with an abnormal ABR demonstrated difficulty with speech discrimination. However, Russolo and Poli (5) reported that the various tests, including pure-tone audiometry, ABR testing, and speech audiometry, were valuable but were not strongly correlated. We reported a correlation with ABR abnormality patterns.

Speech discrimination in previous reports was tested by English or Italian monosyllabic words that carried semantic content. In contrast, Japanese speech audiometry materials are composed of nonsense monosyllabic consonant-vowel units. The Japanese monosyllable tests seem to be more specific to speech perception than English or Italian monosyllable word tests. For this reason the Japanese tests may reveal the effects of lesions in the auditory nerve or brainstem more clearly.

Procedures

Monosyllable Test

A total of 53 consonant-vowel nonsense monosyllables were selected for this discrimination test (Fig. 1). The monosyllables were recorded on a magnetic tape in

Monosyllables									
pa	pi	pɯ	pe	po	ba	bi	bɯ	be	bo
ma	mi	mɯ	me	mo	na	ni	nɯ	ne	no
sa	ʃi	sɯ	se	so					
ta	tʃi	tsɯ	te	to	da	dʒi	dzɯ	de	do
ra	ri	rɯ	re	ro					
					dza			dze	dzo
ka	ki	kɯ	ke	ko	ga	gi	gɯ	ge	go

Fig. 1. List of 53 consonant-vowel nonsense monosyllables

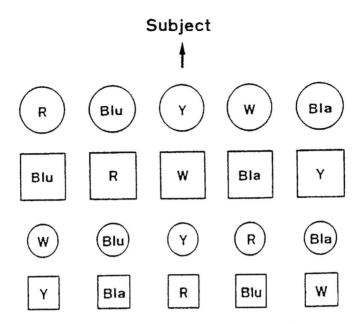

Fig. 2. Arrangement of tokens. *R*, red; *Blu*, blue; *Y*, yellow; *W*, white; *Bla*, black. Each subject received a 39-item Japanese version of the token test consisting of six parts, graded by the length and difficulty of the commands

a young woman's voice and presented monaurally at 50 dB above the patient's subjective threshold (1000 Hz). The percent of correct answers to the 53 nonsense monosyllables test was 84% ± 7% (average patient age 30 years; $n = 20$), and no right–left ear differences were found.

Token Test

The Token test, developed by Renzi and Vignolo (6) for testing auditory comprehension, was given as well. The percent of correct answers to the Token test in normal subjects was 98% ± 3% (average patient age 44.9 years; $n = 54$). All tests were performed in a soundproof room (Fig. 2).

Results

Patients were divided into two major groups according to performance on the monosyllable test. One (group A) consisted of patients with abnormal ABRs and abnormal perception. The other (group B) consisted of patients with abnormal ABRs and normal perception.

Group A: ABR Abnormality and Auditory Abnormal Perception

Type 1: Waves I and II Only

The patients in group A had only waves I and II in the ear on one side (Fig. 3). In case 1, a 10-year-old boy with pontine glioma, the right ABR showed waves I and II only, and the left ABR showed waves I–IV. Pure-tone audiometry revealed slight elevation of the right ear threshold but normal levels in the left ear. The monosyllable test results indicated a mild deficit (1 SD) with the right ear affected more than the left. In case 2, a 46-year-old woman with meningioma at the cerebellopontine angle, the left ABR showed waves I and II only and the right ABR showed waves I–IV with later indistinct waves. Pure-tone audiometry revealed very mild threshold elevation on the right. The monosyllable test disclosed marked impairment of auditory

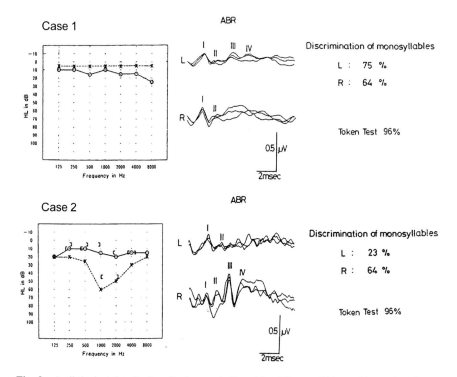

Fig. 3. Audiological data for type 2 of group A. Case 1 is a 10-year-old boy with pontine glioma. Case 4 is a 46-year-old woman with meningioma at the right cerebellopontine angle. In both cases, the auditory brainstem response (*ABR*) of one ear showed waves I and II only. The other ears showed waves I–IV in case 2 and an almost normal response in case 4. In both cases, results of nonsense monosyllable tests were poorer on the side of ABR waves I and II only. In Token tests, both patients showed a normal range

perception on the left side in contrast with the right side. In both cases 1 and 2, the Token test scores were normal. The patients showed unilateral impairment of auditory perception with only waves I and II on the affected side.

Type 2: Waves I, II, and III Only

Other group A patients had waves I, II, and III only on one side (Fig. 4). In case 3, a 40-year-old man with pontine hemorrhage, the left ABR showed only waves I, II, and III, with the right ABR being normal. Although pure-tone audiometry revealed a normal threshold in the speech range, the monosyllable test indicated poorer score performance with the right ear contralateral to the side with the abnormal ABR; the left-side scores were in the normal range. In case 4, a 64-year-old

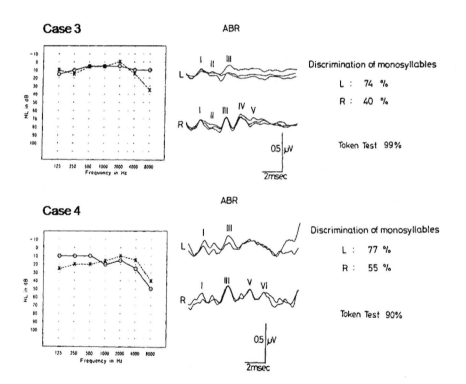

Fig. 4. Audiological data from type 3 of group A. Case 3 is a 40-year-old man with a pontine hemorrhage, and case 4 is a 64-year-old man with a pontine infarction. With pure tone audiometry, both cases showed a near-normal threshold and slight right–left threshold differences. The left ABR of both cases showed waves I, II, and III only whereas the right ABR showed normal waves I–V. Note that results of the nonsense monosyllable test were poorer for the contralateral ear of ABR with waves I, II, and III only

man with a brainstem infarction, the ABR on the left side showed waves I, II, and III only; the right ABR was normal. Although pure-tone audiometry showed a slight threshold increase bilaterally, the monosyllable test revealed a deficit for the right ear again contralateral to the side with the abnormal ABR. Normal performance was shown for the left ear.

Type 3: Prolongation of Wave V-I Peak Interval

Some group A patients showed marked prolongation of the wave V-I peak interval (Fig. 5). Case 5 was a 34-year-old man with a right cerebellopontine angle tumor.

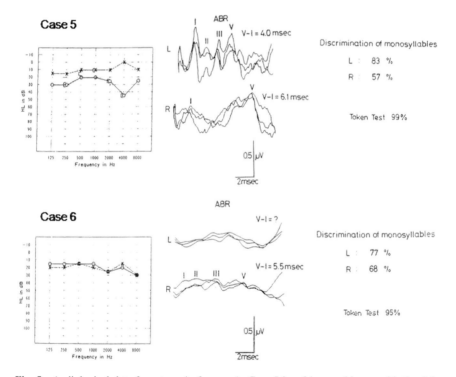

Fig. 5. Audiological data from type 4 of group A. Case 5 is a 34-year-old man with the right cerebellopontine angle tumor, and case 8 is a 62-year-old man with olivopontocerebellar degeneration. In case 5, pure tone threshold is more elevated at the affected ear. The right ABR demonstrated marked prolongation of the wave V-I peak interval, which is more than 3 SD from the normal mean. Note that the results of the nonsense monosyllable test are poorer on the affected side. In case 6, the pure tone audiogram shows a near-normal threshold with no right–left difference. Judgment about the left ABR is reserved because the configuration is unclear; however, the right ABR shows marked prolongation of the wave V-I interval, which is >3 SD from the normal mean latencies. The nonsense monosyllable test showed a lower score on the right side

The ABR of the right, affected side showed a markedly prolonged wave V-I peak interval (which was greater than the 3 SD from the mean in subjects with normal hearing). Pure-tone audiometry showed mild threshold elevation on the affected side, whereas the opposite side had a normal threshold. The monosyllable test scores were lower for the affected side but within the normal range on the unaffected side. The Token test results were in the normal range. In case 6, a 62-year-old man with olivopontocerebellar degeneration wave V-I peak interval, of the right ABR was significantly prolonged more than 3 SD. The left ear ABR could not be evaluated because of its disordered structure.

Pure-tone audiometry showed a slight sensorineural hearing threshold elevation. The monosyllable test showed lower than normal scores for both sides. These two cases suggest that marked prolongation of wave V-I peak latency is related to a decreased capacity for speech perception.

Group B: ABR Abnormality but Normal Auditory Perception

Group B, which showed normal auditory perception despite abnormal ABR configuration, is divided into two subtypes.

Type 1: Wave I Only

Type 1 patients had only wave I bilaterally (Fig. 6). Case 7 was a 28-year-old man with olivopontocerebellar degeneration. In this case a lower brainstem disorder was suspected because of the presence of only wave I. Pure-tone audiometry showed a normal hearing threshold, and the monosyllable test revealed no abnormalities: right (R) 88%, left (L) 91%.

Type 2: Prolongation of Wave V-I Peak Interval

The type 2 patients had bilaterally prolonged wave V-I peak intervals that were more than 2 SD from the normal mean but less than 3 SD. Cases 10–15, which are illustrated in Fig. 6, belong to this subtype. All of the pure-tone audiograms for these patients showed no threshold elevation bilaterally. The monosyllable test scores were in the normal range: case 8 (R 90%, L 90%); case 9 (R 75%, L 76%); case 10 (R 86%, L 93%); case 11 (R 90%, L 92%); case 12 (R 82%, L 78%); case 13 (R 88%, L 85%. Token test results for all were within the normal range.

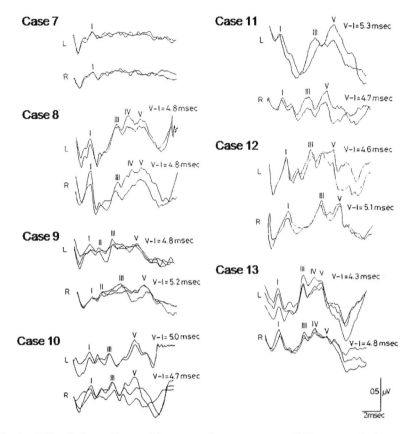

Fig. 6. ABRs of all type B cases. The scores of nonsense monosyllable tests are in the normal range. Case 7 shows only wave I bilaterally. Others show slight prolongation of the wave V-I peak interval, which is more than 2 SD but less than 3 SD

Comment

For the type 1 group A patients, only waves I and II were elicited coincidentally. In the two cases of the group, the scores from the monosyllables tests for the side with waves I and II only were worse than on the other side. This difference of impaired perception might be due to an ipsilateral lesion near the level of the cochlear nucleus. The generator of wave II is presumed to be the cochlear nucleus in cats and the superior olivary complex in humans.

A pattern was observed for the patients of group A in which waves I, II, and III were unilateral. The discrimination of monosyllables was worse in the ear contralateral to the abnormal ABR. Stephens and Thornton (1) found that unilateral abnormalities in low redundancy speech tests were related to contralateral wave V abnormalities on the ABR. The generator of waves IV and V in humans is presumed to be the upper brainstem, which is beyond the decussation at the level of the superior olivary complex. Because those generators are predominantly on the contralateral side of the upper brainstem, it is reasonable that contralateral impairment of scores of monosyllable tests is likely.

In other group A patients, the wave I–II interval was much prolonged. In those two cases, the scores from monosyllable tests were markedly worse on the affected side. Jerger and Jerger (2, 3) reported two similar cases. The patients had normal maximum intelligibility scores with mild rollover. The right ear showed wave I only and normal maximum intelligibility scores without rollover. However, Stephens and Thornton (1) reported that the unilateral abnormalities in low redundancy speech tests were related to ipsilateral wave IV abnormalities.

Some group B patients had only wave I elicited bilaterally, but other audiological data were normal. Jerger and Jerger reported similar cases. In a patient suffering from multiple sclerosis, both ears showed only wave I and normal maximum intelligibility scores for PB word material. Other patients in group B showed bilateral prolongation of the wave interval that was more than 2 SD from the normal mean but less than 3 SD. In these cases, other audiologica; data were completely normal perhaps because the lesions were smaller than those in group A patients.

Scores of the monosyllables tests were impaired in group A but not in group B. However, Musiek and Geurkink (4) reported that speech discrimination ability in patients with abnormal ABR seemed relatively insensitive to brainstem involvement as all scores were good to excellent. Still other authors have reported some abnormalities in speech audiometry, varying from slight to pronounced. This variation in test results is not surprising, considering both the complexity of the central auditory system and the widely variable physiological effects of similar lesions in the central nervous system (CNS) as well as use of different test materials. The present series of patients illustrates this complexity and variability.

Auditory comprehension, which was tested by the Token test, was normal in all the presented cases. These findings imply that the brainstem auditory pathway could play a role in the conduction of speech signal with low redundancy to the higher level, while not affecting auditory comprehension in the presented population. The brainstem auditory pathway with lesions indicated that an abnormal ABR could not always conduct the speech signal of nonsense monosyllables with low redundancy early but could convey meaningful words and sentences. These results imply that brainstem auditory pathway disorders seem to be sensitive to speech units with lower redundancy but not to words or sentences with much more redundancy.

References

1. Stephens SD, Thornton AR (1976) Subjective and electrophysiologic tests in brain stem lesions. Arch Otolaryngol 102:608–613

2. Jerger J, Jerger S (1974) Auditory findings in brain stem disorders. Arch Otolaryngol 99:342–350
3. Jerger S, Jerger J (1975) Extra- and intra-axial brain stem auditory disorders. Audiology 14:93–117
4. Musiek FE, Geurkink NA (1982) Auditory brain stem response and central auditory test findings for patients with brain stem lesions: a preliminary report. Laryngoscope 92:891–899
5. Russolo M, Poli P (1983) Lateralization, impedance, auditory brainstem response and synthetic sentence audiometry in brain stem disorders. Audiology 22:50–62
6. De Renzi E, Vignolo LA (1962) The token test: a sensitive test to detect receptive disturbances in aphasics. Brain 85:665–678

Palatal Myoclonus[2]

Palatal myoclonus (PM) is characterized by continuous, rhythmic involuntary twitching of the oropharyngeal muscles (1). PM is a unique neurological sign due to a brainstem disorder specifically involving Guillain-Mollaret's triangle, which consists of the red nucleus and inferior olivary nuclei. PM has been reported to be frequently associated with various abnormal waveforms of ABRs (2, 3). However, the audiological deficiencies in patients with PM have rarely been studied.

Case Reports

We conducted an investigation of brainstem auditory processing for speech discrimination in three patients.

The patients ranged in age from 40 to 42 years (Figs. 1, 2). Two patients developed PM after pontine hemorrhage. These two patients had ABR abnormalities that correlated with the location of their brainstem lesions despite relatively normal pure-tone threshold tests. Both the nonsense monosyllable test and the dichotic listening test revealed dominance on the side ipsilateral to the lesion, whereas ABR abnormalities were present on the contralateral side. These results suggest that brainstem lesions producing PM could have an effect on auditory perception.

The precise mechanism of PM is unknown, although the responsible lesions have been well defined. These lesions are located on the vertices or sides of a triangle, the "Guillain-Mollaret's triangle" (1), whose vertices are one dentate nucleus of the cerebellum and the contralateral nucleus rubber and inferior olivary nucleus. Moreover, it is known that lesions in this area secondarily cause pseudohypertrophy of the inferior olivary nucleus (2).

---

[2]This section of the chapter was excerpted from: Kurauchi T, Kaga K, Shindo M. Abnormalities of ABR and auditory perception test findings in acquired palatal myoclonus. *Int J Neurosci* 85:273–283, 1996. By permission.

PATIENT 1. 42 M

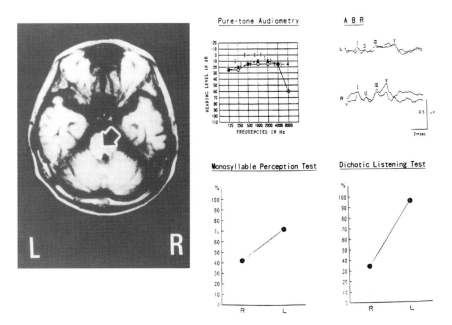

Pure-tone Audiometry

A B R

Monosyllable Perception Test

Dichotic Listening Test

Fig. 1. Magnetic resonance imaging scans of patient 1 show a lesion in the dorsal part of the left pons (*arrow*). Other findings of pure-tone audiometry, the auditory brainstem response (ABR), nonsense monosyllable perception test, and the dichotic listening test are shown as well

PATIENT 2. 40 M

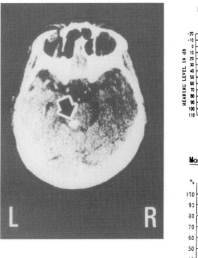

Pure-tone Audiometry

A B R

Monosyllable Perception Test

Dichotic Listening Test

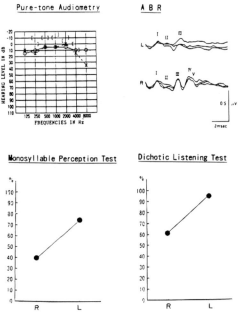

Fig. 2. Computed tomography scan of patient 2 shows a lesion in the dorsal part of the pons on the left side (*arrow*). Pure-tone audiometry, ABR, nonsense monosyllable perception test, and dichotic listening test findings are shown as well

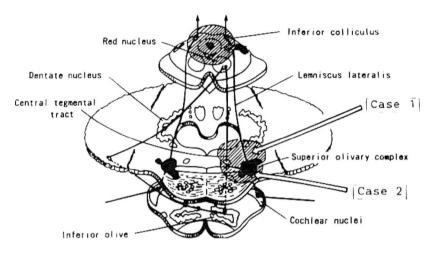

Fig. 3. Suspected loci of the lesions of patients 1 and 2 (*open arrows*) relative to Guillain-Mollaret's triangle and the auditory brainstem pathway

Comment

Because Guillain-Mollaret's triangle is located close to the auditory brainstem pathway, abnormal ABRs have often been reported in patients with PM (2, 3). The pattern of ABR abnormalities varies depending on the location of the lesion. In the present study, two patients showed abnormal ABRs but the pattern of the abnormalities differed among the cases. The III–V interval was prolonged unilaterally in patient 1 and the V wave was absent unilaterally in patient 2. The V wave amplitude was decreased bilaterally, and no abnormalities were detected in the brainstem on the image except pseudohypertrophy of the bilateral inferior olivary nuclei. However, it is highly possible that a lesion existed in the midbrain, considering the pattern of ABR abnormalities. The suspected loci of the lesions in each of our two patients are illustrated in relation to Guillain-Mollaret's triangle and the auditory brainstem pathway in Fig. 3.

We noted a possible relation between the location of brainstem damage and the degree of hearing disturbance. The two patients did not report any hearing problems. This difference in symptoms should be reflected in the severity or location of the damage to the auditory brainstem pathway.

References

1. Turazzi A, Alexandre A, Bricolo A, et al (1977) Opsoclonus and palatal myoclonus during prolonged post-traumatic coma. Eur Neurol 15:257–263

2. Westmoreland BF, Sharbrought FW, Stockard JJ, et al (1983) Brainstem auditory evoked potentials in 20 patients with palatal myoclonus. Arch Neurol 40:155–158
3. Ebstein CM, Stappenbeck R, Karp HR (1980) Brainstem auditory evoked responses in palatal myoclonus. Ann Neurol 7:592

ABR Changes in Pediatric Brainstem Diseases

There can be few things more heartbreaking than deterioration of a previously healthy infant or child. The following five reports detail the changes in the ABR that are seen with five degenerative disorders. Note the behavioral audiometric findings—there can be profound changes in the ABR with preservation of auditory sensitivity.

Adrenoleukodystrophy[3]

Adrenoleukodystrophy (ALD) is a progressive metabolic disease that results in rapid degeneration of the central nervous system (CNS) (1). Both demyelination of white matter and hypermyelination of gray matter in the cerebrum have been associated with ALD (2). Initially, loss of hearing and/or vision are usually observed. The disease progresses rapidly to a decerebrate state in its terminal stage.

Because ALD progresses rapidly resulting in profound neurological deficits, it is difficult to locate lesions as they develop. The auditory evoked response offers a noninvasive method for assessing localized brain function, and the test procedure is simple and fast. For these reasons, the auditory evoked response is ideally suited to evaluate the course of ALD (3).

Case Report

Serial studies of auditory brainstem evoked responses (ABRs) and slow vertex responses (SVRs) were obtained during the progress of ALD in a 6-year-old boy. This child was normal until 5 years of age. His illness began with a gait disturbance, dysarthria, and hearing difficulty (Fig. 1). Later, spastic paralysis, serious deafness, and blindness appeared. He died of respiratory failure 2 years after the onset.

The ABR was normal at onset but changed to an abnormal pattern. Initially, there was lengthening of the wave V-I interpeak interval (Fig. 2), followed by disappearance of the later components as his general condition deteriorated. At the terminal stage, only a prolonged wave I was recordable. The postmortem pathology of the brain revealed demyelination of auditory nerves and marked neuronal loss in the auditory pathways of the brainstem (Figs. 3, 4); in addition, there was a

---

[3]This section of the chapter was excerpted from: Kaga K, Tokoro Y, Tanaka Y, Ushijima H. The progress of adrenoleukodystrophy as revealed by auditory brainstem evoked responses and brainstem histology. *Arch Otorhinolaryngol* 228:17–27, 1980.

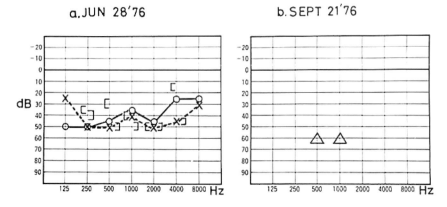

Fig. 1. *Left* Audiogram by play audiometry at the first visit. *Right* Three months later. Thresholds were determined by behavioral observation audiometry

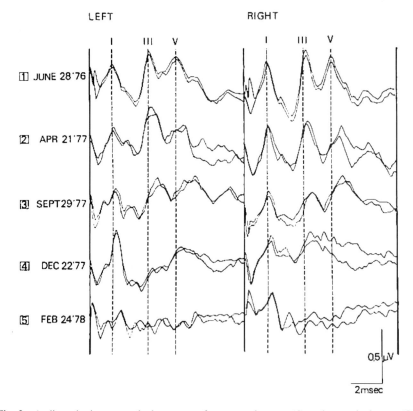

Fig. 2. Auditory brainstem evoked responses from an early stage (*1*) to the terminal stage (*5*)

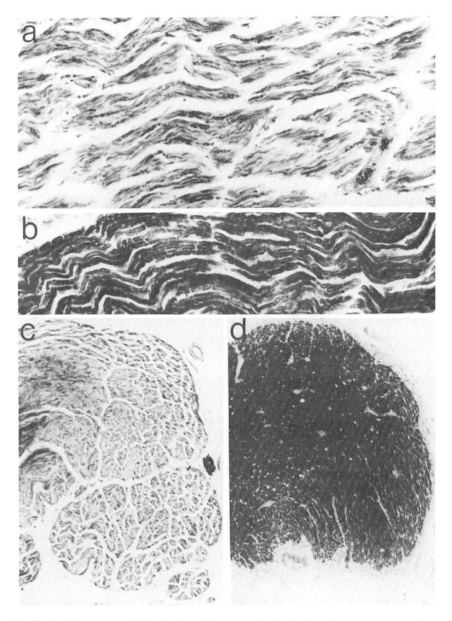

Fig. 3. Auditory nerves. Histologically, VIII nerves (**a** longitudinal section; **c** transverse section) are demyelinated, but facial nerves (**b** longitudinal section; **d** transverse section) are not damaged. (Luxol fast blue-cresyl violet stain. Longitudinal sections ×40, transverse sections ×100)

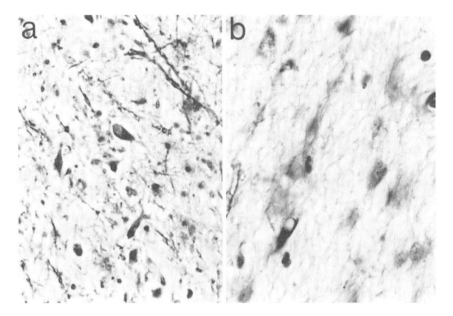

Fig. 4. Cochlear nucleus. **a** Most of the ganglionic nerve cells in the dorsal cochlear nucleus are lost, and the nerve fibers are demyelinated. **b** Most of the ganglionic nerve cells in the ventral cochlear nucleus are severely atrophic, and some of them contain vacuoles. (**a, b** Luxol fast blue-cresyl violet stain. **a** ×100, **b** ×200)

variety of extensive degeneration throughout the cerebrum, particularly complete degeneration of white matter with secondarily occurring ganglionic cell changes. These data suggest that degeneration of the brainstem from rostral to caudal levels occurred.

Comment

This study also illustrates an important capability of ABRs. Not only can they help identify the location of lesions (3), they can be used to evaluate the progress of degenerative diseases such as ALD.

References

1. Allen N, Sherard ES Jr (1975) Developmental and degenerative disease of the brain. In: Farmer RW (eds) Pediatric neurology, 2nd edition. Harper & Row, Hagerstown, MD, pp 118–221
2. Schaumburg JJ, Powers JM, Raine CS, et al (1975) Adrenoleucodystrophy: a clinical and pathologic study of 17 cases. Arch Neurol 32:577–591
3. Ochs R, Markand ON, DeMyer WE (1979) Brainstem auditory evoked responses in leukodystrophies. Neurology 29:1089–1093

Pelizaeus-Merzacher Disease[4]

Pelizaeus reported the first case of Pelizaeus-Merzacher disease (PMD) in 1885 (1). PMD, an X-linked recessive inheritance disease, manifests as dysmyelination in the CNS and is regarded as a kind of leukodystrophy in neuropathology (2, 3). However, PMD has been rarely reported from the viewpoints of otology and neurootology.

Pelizaeus-Merzacher disease is classified into six types. Patients with type II PMD show congenital nystagmus, hypotonia, rigidity of the trunk and extremities, and mental and speech retardation as the main clinical symptoms (3). The pathological features of PMD are as follows.

- Myelin islets or an area of preserved myelin sheath in islet form, called "tigroid" that is located most typically in the gray matter of the cerebrum in autopsy specimens
- Few myelin degenerative products
- No dysmyelination in the spinal root of cranial nerves or in peripheral nerves
- Preserved axons in the dysmyelinated area

Several studies have pointed out that mutations in the proteolipid protein (PLP) gene on the X chromosome are causes of PMD (4).

After objective audiometry of the ABR was introduced in 1970, it was found that only waves I and II of the ABR configuration were detected in PMD pediatric patients (5–9) (Fig. 1). However, hearing, speech, and language abilities of PMD adult patients have not been well studied.

This disease, thought to be a dysmyelinating disorder of the brain that begins during the prenatal period, is caused by some gene mutations. It manifests as horizontal nystagmus and severe rigidity of the extremities (Fig. 2).

Among the five patients studied here, one patient's T2-weighted MRI scans revealed a high signal of the white matter and a low signal of the gray matter in the cerebrum, but there were no abnormal intensities of either area in the cerebellum or the spinal cord (Fig. 3). Although such patients show only waves I and II in the ABR, they have relatively good hearing ability at around 30 dB. They cannot speak words but can hear well and enjoy listening to conversation and music. One of them had a normal hearing threshold in pure-tone audiometry and normal speech discrimination during speech audiometry (Fig. 4). This can be explained by a nerve conduction blockade through dysmyelinated axons or the desynchronization of neurons and nerves in waves following waves I and II (9). At present, the described patients are living with their families as young adults.

---

[4]This section of the chapter was excerpted from: Kaga K, Tamai F, Kodama M, Kodama K. Three young adult patients with Pelizaeus-Merzacher disease who showed only waves I and II in auditory brainstem response but had good auditory perception. *Acta Otolaryngol* 125:1018–1023, 2005. By permission.

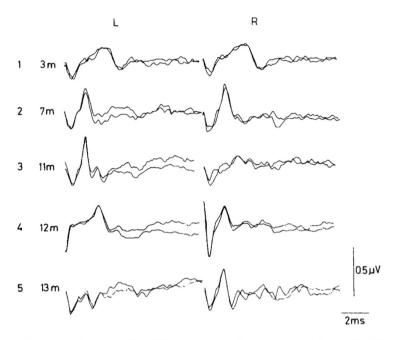

Fig. 1. Only wave I or waves I and II are present in five nystagmus infants with Pelizaeus-Merzacher disease

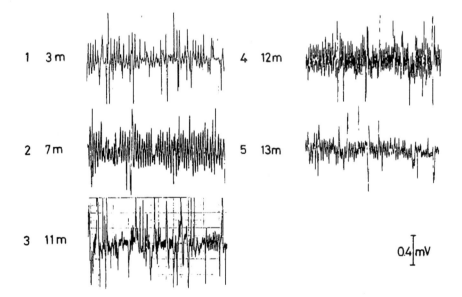

Fig. 2. Spontaneous eye movement recordings of five patients by electronystagmography (time constant 0.003 s) showing typical pendular nystagmus

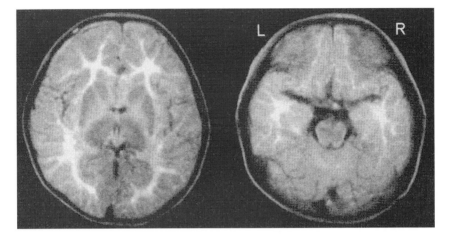

Fig. 3. T2-weighted magnetic resonance imaging (MRI) of the brain shows high-intensity signal in the subcortical area

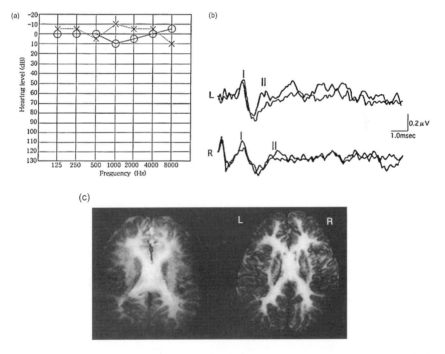

Fig. 4. Case 3. **a** Pure-tone audiometry: normal threshold. **b** Auditory brainstem responses: Only waves I and II are shown. **c.** T2-weighted MRI of the brain shows a high-intensity signal in the subcortical area. This patient showed normal speech discrimination

References

1. Pelizaeus R (1885) Über eine eigent ü mliche Form spasticher Lähmung mit Zerebalerch-
   seinumgen auf hereditärer Grundlage (multiplel Sklerose). Arch Psychiatr Nervenkr
   16:698–710
2. Merezbacher L (1910) Eine eigenartige familiä Erkrankungsform (Aplasia axialis extracorti-
   calis congenital). Z Ges Neurol Psychiatr 3:1–138
3. Allen IV (1984) Pelizaeus-Merzbacher disease. In: Greenfield's neuropathology. 4th edn.
   Edward Arnold, London, pp 371–373
4. Koeppen AH, Ronca NA, Greenfield EA, et al (1987) Defective biosynthesis of proteolipid
   protein in Pelizaeus-Merzbacher disease. Ann Neurol 21:159–170
5. Garg BP, Markand ON, DeMyer WE (1983) Usefulness of BAER studies in the early diagnosis
   of Pelizaeus-Merzbacher disease. Neurology 33:955–956
6. Kaga K, Kitazumi E, Kodama K (1986) Absence of later auditory brainstem response components, congenital horizontal nystagmus and hypotonia in male infants. Ann Otol Rhinol
   Laryngol 95:203–206
7. Wang PJ, Chen RL, Shen YZ (1989) Hypotonia, congenital nystamgus and abnormal auditory
   brainstem response. Pediatr Neurol 5:381–383
8. Kaga M, Murakami T, Naitoh H (1990) Studies on pediatric patients with absent auditory
   brainstem response (ABR) later components. Brain Dev 12:380–384
9. Kaga K, Tamai F, Kodama M, et al (2005) Only waves I and II of auditory brainstem responses
   and auditory perception in three young adult patients with Pelizaeus-Merzbacher disease. Acta
   Otolaryngol 125:1018–1023

Infantile Gaucher's Disease[5]

Gaucher's disease is classified into three types—those affecting adults, infants, and
juveniles, respectively (1). Infantile Gaucher's disease, called "type 2, acute neu-
ronopathic Gaucher's disease," usually presents within 6 months of birth, the
neonatal period often being normal. The first signs of hepatosplenomegaly, failure
to thrive, or difficulty feeding can occur singly or in combination. Motor delay is
evident by 6 months, and it progresses to cranial nerve and extrapyramidal tract
involvement. Seizures are not common. Death, usually from pulmonary infection,
occurs before the second birthday. The gross appearance of the brain is not abnormal in type 2. However, Lake (1) summarized abnormal microscopic findings of
the brain in type 2 of infantile Gaucher's disease: "In the cerebral cortex there is
no evidence of neuronal storage, and only a mild loss of neurons is seen in layers
3 and 5. Myelination appears normal for age. Free Gaucher's cells are found in the
cortex and perivascularly. In the basal ganglia and brainstem, marked to moderate
neuronophagia and gliosis is evident, while in other neurons there is mild cytoplas-
mic swellings suggesting storage."

---

[5]This section of the chapter was excerpted from: Kaga K, Ono M, Yakumaru K, et al. Brainstem
pathology of infantile Gaucher's disease with only wave I and II of auditory brainstem response.
J Laryngol Otol 112:1069–1073, 1998. By permission.

Kaga M et al. (2) recorded only waves I and II and a small wave III in an infant with infantile Gaucher's disease at 6 months of age and only waves I and II by 8 months of age, although the autopsy showed relative preservation of the nuclei and tracts of the auditory pathways in the brainstem. Lacey and Terplan (3) recorded only waves I, II, and III and soon after only waves I and II in an infant with Gaucher's disease who died at 3 months 1 week of age. The autopsy revealed loss of neuronal cells in the cochlear nucleus and superior olivary nucleus as well as the vestibular nucleus, fasciculus cuneatus, inferior olivary nucleus, and dentate nucleus.

Case Report

We studied the ABR and neuropathology in a female infant who died at 6 months of age because of typical infantile Gaucher's disease. The patient was hospitalized for hepatosplenomegaly and failure to thrive. Her ABR showed only waves I and II (Fig. 1).

The neuropathological study disclosed that Gaucher's cells were found in the perivascular region of the cerebrum and anterior ventral nucleus of the thalamus (Fig. 2), and gliosis was found in the dorsal part of the brainstem but not in the ventral part (Fig. 3). 3) Neuronal cells in the superior olivary nucleus were lost, and marked gliosis was found in the cochlear nucleus (Fig. 4). The disappearance of wave III and later waves of ABR were supported by the pathological findings (4).

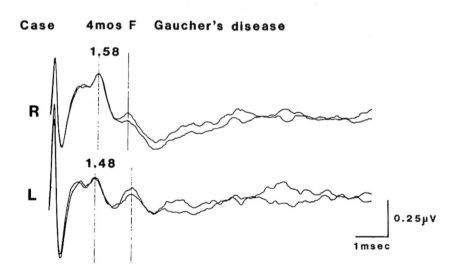

Fig. 1. Auditory brainstem response at 4 months of age. Only waves I and II were elicited in both ears. *R*, right; *L*, left

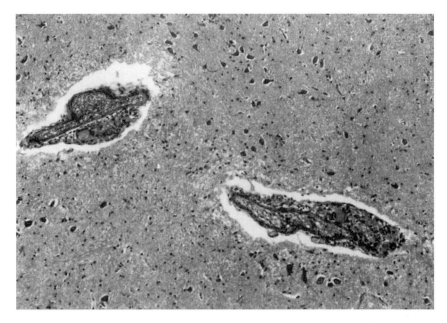

Fig. 2. Large Gaucher's cells in the anterior ventral nucleus of the thalamus. (H&E, ×100)

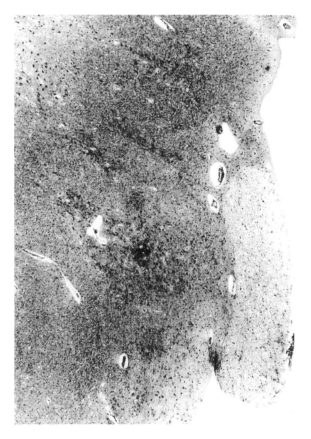

Fig. 3. Gliosis in the cochlear nerve (*CN*) and the cochlear nucleus. *VCN*, ventral cochlear nucleus; *DCN*, dorsal cochlear nucleus. (H&E, ×40)

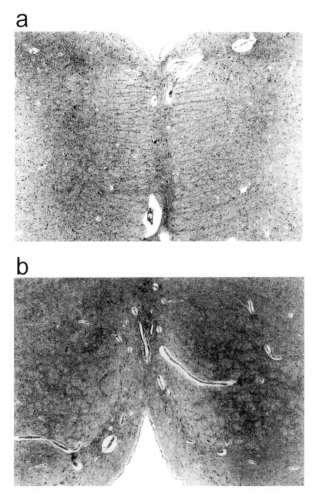

Fig. 4. Cross section of lower brainstem. Gliosis was more marked in the dorsal part (**a**) than in the ventral part (**b**). Note also the loss of neuronal cells in the superior olivary nucleus. *SON*, superior olivary nucleus; *DCN*, dorsal cochlear nucleus. (H&E, ×4)

Comment

In our patient, the location of lesions clearly included the lower brainstem, as shown in the neuropathology and by the ABR, which demonstrated only waves I and II without subsequent waves. Similar abnormal configurations of the ABRs have been reported in patients with lower brainstem neurological diseases. In lesion studies and field analysis in animal experiments, the origins of waves I and II were demonstrated to be the ipsilateral auditory nerve and cochlear nucleus. The origins of wave III were reported to be the bilateral superior olivary complexes. These reports of the origins of the ABR in clinical and animal studies predict involvement of the projections to the olivary complexes or the nuclei themselves in our case.

Finally, it is noted that the ABR abnormality was well correlated with brainstem pathology in our case. We emphasize that the ABR is a useful tool for evaluating brainstem function and pathology in infantile Gaucher's disease if the brainstem involvement exists in the brainstem auditory pathway. It is quite possible to have a normal ABR in some early cases. On the other hand, ABR latencies can be useful in some cases to look at involvement of the auditory pathways, and serial ABRs may be helpful for assessing the progress of the disease.

References

1. Lake BD (1984) Infantil Gaucher's disease. In: Adames JH, Corsellis JAN, Duchen LW (eds) Gaucher disease. 4th edn. Edward Arnold, London, pp 522–526
2. Kaga M, Azuma C, Imamura T, et al (1982) Auditory brainstem response (ASBR) in infantile Gaucher's disease. Neuropediatrics 13:207–210
3. Lacey DJ, Terplan K (1984) Correlating auditory evoked and brainstem histological abnormalities in infantile Gaucher's disease. Neurology 34:539–541
4. Kaga K, Ono M, Yakumaru K, et al (1998) Brainstem pathology of infantile Gaucher's disease with only wave I and II of auditory brainstem response. J Laryngol Otol 112:1069–1073

Cockayne's Syndrome[6]

Cockayne's syndrome (CS) is a rare autosomal recessive, premature aging disorder that is clinically characterized by dwarfism, mental retardation, microcephaly, ataxia, pigmentary degeneration of the retina, progeroid features, photosensitivity, and sensorineural deafness (1, 2). This syndrome is neuropathologically regarded as a form of leukodystrophy (3).

Hearing disorder is one of the major clinical features of CS. Usually, hearing impairment becomes apparent during the course of the disease and progresses as the patient deteriorates neurologically, but the progress of hearing loss in CS has not been confirmed neuropathologically or neurophysiologically. The hearing disorder in CS is considered to be sensorineural in origin (4), but the site of the lesion

---

[6]This section of the chapter was excerpted from: Iwasaki S, Kaga K, Yagi M, Kuroda M. Vestibular findings and brainstem pathology in two siblings with Cockayne's syndrome. *ORL J Otorhinolarygol Relat Spec* 58:343–346, 1996. By permission.

causing hearing loss is unclear. In our study, the ABRs showed gross abnormalities in all four patients with CS, suggesting widespread demyelination of the brainstem (5). CS is considered to be a form of leukodystrophy. The most common neuro-pathological findings are severe microcephaly, central white matter atrophy with patchy demyelination, and calcification of the basal ganglia (6, 7).

Case Reports

Case 1

A male infant was born after a normal pregnancy at 41 gestational weeks; he weighed 2832 g at birth. His parents are cousins, and he is their only child. His early developmental milestones were reached normally, but subsequent develop-ment was delayed. He sat at 10 months of age and crawled at 12 months. He was unable to walk without aid. His limbs were stiff, and there was limitation of move-ment of various joints. He was always extremely sensitive to sunlight. At 2 years of age, he showed less than average height and weight for his age (72.8 cm, 8120 g) and microcephaly (head circumference 42.8 cm). His facial appearance, with a beaked nose and sunken eyes, was characteristic of CS. He was mentally retarded and could not say any meaningful words. Funduscopic examination revealed bilat-eral "salt and pepper" retinal pigmentation and retinal artery narrowing but no optic atrophy. Brain computed tomography (CT) revealed calcification of the bilateral basal ganglia and dilatation of the ventricles. At 13 years of age, he still could not walk without help or say more than a few words. The chronological findings of pure-tone audiometry and ABR testing showed progression of brainstem lesion and sensory neural hearing loss (Fig. 1).

Case 2

A male infant was born at full term after an uneventful pregnancy. The birth weight was 2750 g, length 50 cm, and head circumference 33.5 cm. His maternal grand-father and paternal grandmother were cousins. Two of the four siblings exhibited signs of this syndrome, whereas the remaining two are normal. The developmental milestones for the patient were abnormal: he sat at 9 months, crawled at 11 months, and walked with aid at 18 months. He was unable to walk without help at any time during his life. He could say a few single words at the age of 4 years, but speech did not develop thereafter. Hearing loss was noted at the age of 5 years, and he had begun to use bilateral hearing aids. His gait disturbance progressed after the age of 9 years.

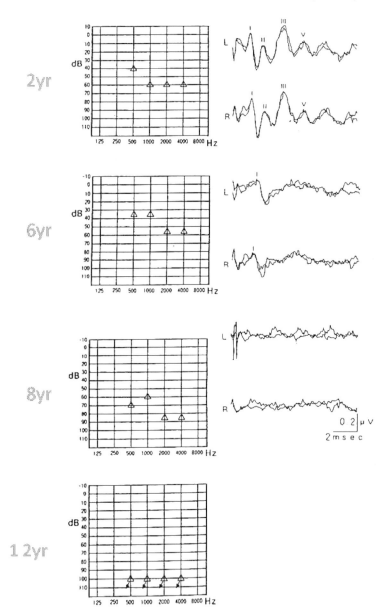

Fig. 1. Case 1. *Left* Thresholds determined by conditioned orientation reflex (COR) audiometry at the age of 2, 6, 8, and 12 years. *Right* Auditory brainstem responses at the age of 2, 6, and 8 years

On physical examination at 11 years of age, his height and weight were lower than average for his age (86.4 cm, 7.3 kg), and he exhibited microcephaly. His facial appearance was peculiar, with a beaked nose, sunken eyes, and prominent maxilla. His teeth were highly carious. He was mentally retarded and could not say any meaningful words. Neurological examination revealed truncal ataxia, with intention tremor of all four extremities. He walked from object to object for support. The gait was wide-based, slow, and unsteady. There was no paralysis of the external ocular muscles. Nystagmus was not evident in the primary position, but he had horizontal gaze-evoked nystagmus on right and left lateral gaze. Funduscopic examinations showed bilateral "salt and pepper" retinal pigmentation. The scores for conditioned orientation reflex audiometry were off the scale at all frequencies. Click-evoked ABRs were absent at 95 dB nHL in both ears. Brain CT revealed calcification of the bilateral basal ganglia and dilatation of the ventricles. In the damped-rotation test, no vestibular nystagmus was observed in either clockwise or counterclockwise rotations.

He died of pneumonia at the age of 15 years. Autopsy was performed 4 h after his death.

Neuropathological findings indicated that the weight of the whole brain was 340 g. The cerebral while matter was reduced, and the ventricles were enlarged. The substantia nigra was deeply pigmented, the corpus callosum was thin, and the cerebellum was symmetrically atrophic. The brainstem was attenuated at all levels. Histologically, the cerebral white mater revealed irregular patchy demyelination in all areas. There were basophilic calcospherites in the basal ganglia. In the cerebellum, there was diffuse neuronal loss throughout the molecular, ganglionic, and granular layers with Bergmann gliosis. The remaining Purkinje cells were disaligned, and the granular layer contained many torpedoes. The dentate nucleus was markedly degenerated. Patchy demyelination and diffuse fibrillary gliosis, predominantly in the tegmentum, were present throughout the brainstem. The oculomotor, trochlear, and abducens nuclei appeared normal. The paramedian pontine reticular formation, which is assumed to be located in the medial part of the nucleus reticularis magnocellularis, showed no obvious loss of neurons, although proliferation of glia was found (Fig. 2). The vestibular nuclei showed neuronal loss with fibrillary gliosis. The perihypoglossal nucleus was preserved.

Comment

In CS, demyelination of the brainstem seems to precede that of the cochlear nerve and vestibular nerve. The finding that wave I is generated within the most distal portion of the VIII nerve suggests that the lesion causing hearing loss in CS is in both the central and peripheral brainstem. However, it is unclear whether the lesion causing hearing loss in CS is in the inner ear or at the junction between the VIII nerve and the inner ear (6). Further studies are required to clarify the site of the lesion causing hearing loss in CS.

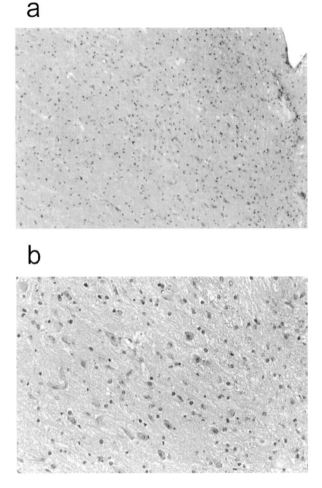

Fig. 2. Pontine reticular formation. **a** Proliferation of glia is evident in the medial portion of the pontine tegmentum. **b** Preservation of the neurons is seen in the medial portions of the nucleus gigantocellularis. (**a**, **b** H&E. **a** ×40, **b** ×100)

References

1. Cockayne EA (1936) Dwarfism with retinal atrophy and deafness. Arch Dis Child 11:1–8
2. Cockayne EA (1946) Case reports: dwarfism with retinal atrophy and deafness. Arch Dis Child 21:52–54
3. Smits MG, Gableels FJM, Reiner WO, et al (1982) Peripheral and central myelinopathy in Cockayne's syndrome. Neuropediatrics 13:161–167
4. Shemen LJ, Mitchell DP, Farkashidy J (1984) Cockayne syndrome—an audiologic and temporal bone analysis. Am J Otol 5:300–307
5. Iwasaki S, Kaga K (1994) Chronological changes of auditory brainstem responses in Cockayne's syndrome. Int J Pediatr Otorhinolaryngol 30:211–221

6. Iwasaki S, Kaga K, Yagi M, et al (1996) Vestibular findings and brainstem pathology in two siblings with Cockayne's syndrome. ORL J Otorhinolaryngol Relat Spec 58:343–346
7. Sugarman GI, Landing BH, Reed WB (1977) Cockayne syndrome: clinical study of two patients and neuropathologic findings in one. Clin Pediatr 16:25–232

Leigh's Syndrome[7]

Leigh's subacute necrotizing encephalomyopathy was first described in 1951 (1). It is now thought to be a heterogeneous disorder (2) and is classified as a type of mitochondrial encephalomyopathy (MEM). Recent advances in the biochemical approach have produced some confusion in the classification of MEM. MEM with lactic acidosis syndrome (MELAS) has been reported as "cortical Leigh syndrome" and shows low-density areas in the cortex on cranial computed tomography (CCT) (3).

Case Reports

Case 1: Cytochrome C Oxidase Deficiency

Patient 1 was a 4-month-old male infant. At 3 months of age he had an apneic attack that required artificial ventilation. At 7 months his respiration became irregular and then apneic, and he was again placed on a respirator. He was comatose and had frequent seizures. His pupils were miotic and reacted to light sluggishly. Corneal reflexes were lost. Oculocephalic responses were depressed but present. The ABR recorded when he was 5 months of age showed a prominent wave I followed by an ambiguous wave II in both leads (Fig. 1). When he was 7 months old, the abnormalities were present, but the waveforms were slightly improved because of the presence of detectable waves II, II, and V, although his clinical condition had worsened.

Case 2: NADH Coenzyme Q Reductase Deficiency

Patient 2 was a 6-year-old girl who had developed repeated alternating hemiconvulsions and hemiplegias followed by mental and motor deterioration. She often had exudative otitis media. The first ABR recording showed an abnormal wave pattern with prolonged latencies of waves in both leads. Serial recordings showed progressive deterioration of the ABR waveforms (Fig. 2).

---

[7]This section of the chapter was excerpted from: Kaga M, Naitoh H, Nihei K. Auditory brainstem response in Leigh's syndrome. *Acta Pediatr Jpn* 29:254–260.

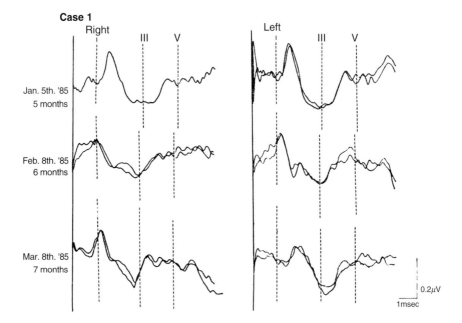

Fig. 1. Case 1. The first ABR showed a prominent wave I and a prolonged later waves in both ears. In the second and third ABRs, the abnormalities were present but the waveforms were somewhat improved; moreover, they did not deteriorate in parallel with the patient's clinical condition

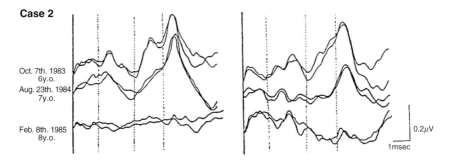

Fig. 2. Case 2. The first ABR showed an abnormal wave pattern, with prolonged latencies of waves in both leads. Serial recordings showed progressive deterioration of the ABRs

Comment

Kaga M et al. (4) reported serial ABRs in eight patients with clinically diagnosed Leigh's syndrome. ABR abnormalities were detected in the early stages of the disease in all patients. A severely abnormal wave configuration associated with prolonged wave latency was detected in patients with apnea and/or other symptomatology involving the brainstem. Patients with cortical involvement had markedly abnormal ABRs in which only waves I and/or V were present. In those patients whose clinical symptoms were less severe, the ABR was mildly abnormal. Changes in the ABR did not consistently reflect the clinical exacerbations and remissions. It has been suggested that ABRs in degenerative diseases are more apt to be abnormal with a white matter disease than with a gray matter disease. In Leigh's syndrome, there is some preference for gray matter, but the borders of the lesions meander across gray and white matter (3). Therefore, we can expect ABR abnormalities in Leigh's syndrome. ABRs were useful in the classification of Leigh's syndrome and in judging the severity of the disease process. ABRs can be used as a supplementary diagnostic procedure for Leigh's syndrome.

References

1. Leigh D (1951) Subacute necrotizing encephalomyelopathy in an infant. J Neurol Neurosurg Psychiatry 14:216–221
2. Sander J, Packman S, Berg BV, et al (1984) Pyruvate carboxylase activity in subacute necrotizing encephalopathy (Leigh's disease). Neurology 34:515–516
3. Egger J, Pincott JR, Wilson J, Erdohazi M (1984) Cortical subacute necrotizing encephalomyelopathy: a study of two patients with mitochondrial dysfunction. Neuropediatrics 15:150–158
4. Kaga M, Naitoh H, Nihei K (1987) ABR in Leigh's syndrome. Acta Pediatr Jpn 29:254–260

Hypoxia and Anoxia[8]

We turn from the often insidious degenerative disease of childhood to the sequelae of acute episodes of anoxia or hypoxia.

It has been reported that age can influence the pattern of the ischemic alterations of the brain due to anoxic or hypoxic accidents (1). Hypoxic brain damage in fetuses and newborns accounts for a high proportion of children with cerebral palsy, mental retardation, epilepsy, and sensory neural hearing loss (1, 2). After the perinatal period, anoxic or hypoxic brain damage sometimes occurs in infants and children due to accidents involving near-suffocation or near-drowning. We report on a study of behavioral audiometry and ABRs in infants and children who were involved in sudden near-suffocation or near-drowning accidents.

The sudden accidents were caused by airway obstruction due to near-drowning in a bathtub, washing machine, river, pond, or pool. Most of the patients suffered cardiac arrest and were subsequently resuscitated.

---

[8]This section of the chapter was excerpted from: Kaga K, Ichimura K, Kitazumi E, et al. Auditory brainstem responses in infants and children with anoxic brain damage due to near-suffocation or near-drowning. *Int J Pediatr Otorhinolaryngol* 36:231–239, 1996.

Case Reports

We studied ABRs of 16 infants and children with brain damage after anoxic accidents due to near-suffocation or near-drowning (Tables 1, 2). The patients manifested cerebral palsy, mental retardation, and/or epilepsy and showed poor responses during behavioral audiometry (Table 3).

Auditory brainstem responses were abnormal in five of the patients in the near-drowning group—waves I, II, and III only were present in three patients, and the amplitudes of waves IV and V were low in two patients (Fig. 1)—but normal in most of the patients in the near-suffocation group. Severe cerebral palsy in six

Table 1. Patients with near-suffocation accidents

Case	Sex	Age at accident	Cause of accident
1	F	2 months	Milk taking
2	M	3 months	Sleeping on a futon[a]
3	M	4 months	Sleeping on a futon
4	M	4 months	Sleeping on a futon
5	M	6 months	Sleeping on a futon
6	F	8 months	Sleeping on a futon
7	F	7 months	General anesthesia
8	F	8 years	General anesthesia

[a] Japanese bedding

Table 2. Patients with near-drowning accidents

Case	Sex	Age at accident	Location of accident
1	M	11 months	Bathtub
2	M	13 months	Bathtub
3	M	19 months	Pond
4	F	2 years	Washing machine filled with water
5	M	2 years	Pond
6	F	3 years	Pool
7	M	5 years	River
8	F	6 years	Bathtub

Table 3. Patients of near-suffocation accidents

Case	Age at examination	Neurological findings	Behavioral auditory (dB HL)	ABR
1	13 months	Cerebral palsy, cortical blindness	No response	Normal
2	3 months	Cerebral palsy	No response	Normal
3	2 years	Cerebral palsy	COR: 90 dB	Normal
4	4 months	Epilepsy, cortical blindness	COR: 45 dB	Normal
5	8 months	Cortical deafness	No response	Normal
6	16 months	Epilepsy, cortical blindness, left microtia, aural atresia	No response	R: normal L: no response
7	10 months	Epilepsy, cortical blindness	No response	Normal
8	9 years	Cerebral palsy, cortical blindness	No response	Normal

ABR, auditory brainstem response; dB HL, decibels hearing level; COR, conditioned orientation reflex audiometry; R, right; L, left

Near-drowning

Case 2 1 yr 4mo

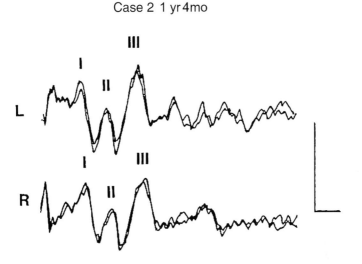

Fig. 1. Typical auditory brainstem responses (ABRs) of the near-suffocation group. Behavior observation audiometry showed no response, although the ABR was normal. *R*, right ear stimulus; *L*, left ear stimulus

Table 4. Patients of near-drowning

Case	Age at examination	Neurological findings	Auditory behavioral audiometry	ABR
1	14 months	Cerebral palsy	No response	Normal
2	16 months	Cerebral palsy	No response	R: waves I, II, III L: waves I, II, III
3	2 years	Cerebral palsy	60 dB	Normal
4	2 years	Cerebral palsy	No response	R: waves I, II, III L: waves I, II, III
5	3 years	Cerebral palsy	No response	R and L: low amplitudes of waves IV, V
6	5 years	Cerebral palsy	No response	R: waves I, II, III L: waves I, II, III
7	6 years	Pseudobulbar palsy, epilepsy	Normal	R and L: low amplitudes of waves IV, V
8	7 years	Epilepsy	Normal	Normal

patients and epilepsy in two patients were associated with mental retardation. Auditory behavioral audiometry showed no responses in six patients but normal responses in two patients. Moreover, ABRs were abnormal in five patients: waves I, II, and III only were present in three patients; and the amplitudes of waves IV and V were low in two patients.

These auditory behavioral audiometry results and ABRs for the near-drowning subjects are summarized in Table 4.

Comment

This difference in the ABRs between the two groups suggest that anoxic brain damage due to near-drowning might involve not only the cerebral cortex and sub-cortical white matter but also the upper brainstem and midbrain in infants and children.

It was reported that the CNS was severely damaged in children due to near-drowning and that prognostic factors were age, duration of hypoxia, time elapsed until resuscitation, coma level, pH of blood gases, and degrees of CT abnormality (3–5). In the cases reported here, the neurological signs were various, possibly because of variation among the cases in the prognostic factors present. Finally, we observed no auditory behavioral response in many of the patients in the near-suffocation group or in the near-drowning group. The absence of these responses (but not peripheral hearing loss) probably resulted from cortical and subcortical brain damage.

References

1. Briererley JB, Graham DI (1984) Cerebral hypoxia. In: Adams JH, Corsellis JAN, Duchen LW (eds) Greenfield's neuropathology. Edward Arnold, London, pp 125–297
2. Hecox K, Cone B (1981) Prognostic importance of auditory evoked responses after asphyxia. Neurology 31:1429–1433
3. Murray RR, Kapia A, Blanco E, et al (1984) Cerebral computed tomography in drowning victims. AJNR Am J Neuroradiol 5:176–179
4. Orlowski JP (1979) Prognostic factors in pediatric cases and the near-drowning. J Am Coll Emerg Physicians 8:176–179
5. Taylor SB, Quencer RM, Holzman BH, et al (1985) Central nervous system anoxic-ischemic insult in children due to near-drowning. Radiology 156:641–646

Midbrain Lesions and Perception[9]

The inferior colliculus (ICs) are important generators of wave V in human ABRs. The following case report describes auditory impairment following surgical removal of a pinealoma. However, pinealomas themselves can cause so-called midbrain deafness, the same disorder as IC deafness.

Siebenmann (1) reported the first case of midbrain deafness in 1896 (Table 1). In the modern age, CT and MRI have demonstrated the location of lesions in patients with a pinealoma to be the inferior colliculus (1–8) (Table 1). We studied a patient with pinealoma whose findings resulted from damage of the IC.

---

[9]This section of the chapter was excerpted from: Yamada K, Kaga K, et al. A case of pinealoma postoperatively presenting with a hearing disorder, downward gaze paralysis, and convergence nystagmus (in Japanese). Audiol Jpn 60:1101–1107, 1988.

Table 1. Reports of hearing disorders in patients with a pinealoma

Year	Author	Description
1896	Siebenmann	Glioma, total deafness of both ears
1925	Horrax & Bailey	Five of fifteen cases showed mild deafness
1932	Harris & Cairns	Hearing improvement after extirpation of a pinealoma
1936	Brunner	One case showed bilateral profound deafness, and another case showed left profound hearing loss
1947	Sloane et al.	Sudden and complete deafness
1957	Kirikae	Bilateral hearing loss; it was worse on the left. Autopsy demonstrated a right MGB lesion
1981	Jerger	Decreased speech perception of the left ear due to a right pineloma
1988	Yamada et al.	Poor speech discrimination; right and left ear difference shown by the dichotic listening test

MGB, medial geniculate body

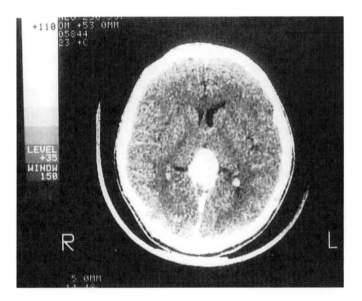

Fig. 1. Computed tomography of the brain in the patient, who had a pinealoma. Slice level of the midbrain and the upper thalamus

Case Report

Postoperative neurological signs in a 22-year-old man with a pinealoma were studied (Fig. 1). After surgical removal of the pinealoma, he suffered from hearing disorder and had difficulty looking downward. An audiological examination disclosed normal thresholds by pure-tone audiometry, normal ABRs and middle-latency responses (MLRs), but abnormally low speech discrimination in both ears

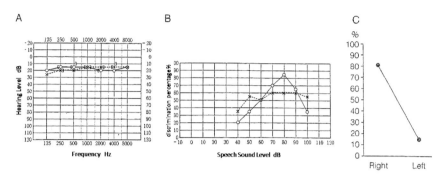

Fig. 2. Auditory examination of patient 1, who had a pinealoma (Fig 1). **A** Normal pure-tone audiogram. **B** Impairment of the speech reception threshold. **C** Marked right and left difference of the dichotic listening test, indicating a left ear disadvantage

(Fig. 2). Neuropsychological examination demonstrated normal auditory comprehension. However, the dichotic listening test demonstrated a marked left ear disadvantage. Eye movement tests showed downward gaze paralysis, lateral gaze nystagmus, and convergence nystagmus. An MRI study revealed a well-defined low-intensity area at the level of the dorsal midbrain.

Comment

It was thought that these signs could be produced by the lesion, which was probably caused by hemorrhage at the operation. It has been postulated that the central nucleus of the IC passes a pure tone of the upper auditory pathway and is concerned with sound localization and generating ABR waves IV and V. However, the function of the IC is not clear. Based on the audiological findings and the MRI scans, we suggest that the cortex of the IC plays an important role in speech discrimination.

References

1. Siebenmann F (1896) Über die zentrale 'Höbahn u. über ihre Schädigung durch Geschwülste des Mittelhirns specielle der Vierhügelgssesgends u. der Haube. Z Ohrenheilk 29:28–91
2. Horrax G, Bailey P (1925) Tumors of the pineal body. Arch Neurol Psychiatry 13:423–435
3. Harris W, Cairns H (1932) Diagnosis and treatment of pineal tumors. Lancet 1:3–15
4. Brunner H (1936) Otologische Diagnostik desr Hirntumoren. Urban Schwarzenberg, Berlin, pp 345–451
5. Sloane P, Persky A, Saltzman M (1943) Midbrain deafness: tumor of the midbrain producing sudden and complete deafness. Arch Neurol Psychiatry 49:237–243

6. Kirikae I (1957) A case of midbrain deafness due to pinealoma. Nippon Jibiinkoka Gakkai Kaiho 60:1357–1367
7. Jerger S (1981) Intracranial tumors affecting the central auditory system. In: Jerger S, Jerger J (eds) Auditory disorders. Little Brown, Boston, pp 79–93
8. Yamada, Kaga K, Shindo M, et al (1988) A case of pinealoma postoperatively presenting with hearing disorder, downward gaze paralysis and convergence nystagmus. Jibika (Tokyo) 60:1101–1107

6
Unilateral Auditory Radiation and/or Auditory Cortex Lesions and Perception

The purpose of this chapter is to evaluate auditory central processing in patients with unilateral auditory radiation or auditory cortex lesions using nonsense monosyllables for speech discrimination, the dichotic listening test, and the Token test for auditory comprehension.

Unilateral Lesions and Auditory Perception

Unilateral lesions of the auditory cortex or auditory radiation are caused by cerebrovascular accidents in the temporal lobe or subcortical area or in the basal ganglia (Figs. 1, 2). Generally, patients do not complain of hearing problems, and even people around them do not detect their disordered hearing. It is possible, however, to reveal perceptual hearing problems using deep neuropsychological testing. Two typical cases are presented in Figs. 1 and 2. Figure 1 shows results from a 57-year-old man with a lesion in the left auditory cortex and radiation after left putaminal hemorrhage. The results clearly demonstrated that the right ear performance is worse than that of the left ear. Figure 2 shows the results from a 37-year-old man with a lesion of the right auditory cortex and radiation after hemorrhage due to an arteriovenous (AV) malformation in the right hemisphere. It is clearly demonstrated that the left ear performance is worse than that of the right ear. There is particularly abnormal audition in the unilateral temporal lobe, including word deafness or melody deafness, caused by the left primary and secondary auditory cortex lesion. Here we summarize the influence of the unilateral temporal lobe lesion on auditory perception.

- Discrimination of nonsense monosyllables was significantly poorer in the ear contralateral to the auditory cortex or auditory radiation lesion than in the ipsilateral ear (Fig. 3).

Central Auditory Pathway Disorders. K. Kaga
doi: 978-4-431-26920-5_6, © Springer 2009

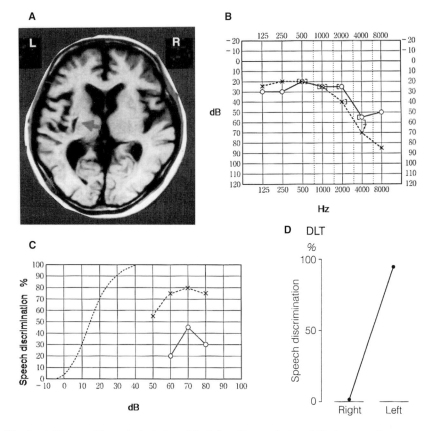

Fig. 1. A 57-year-old man had a lesion of the left auditory radiation. **A** Brain magnetic resonance imaging shows an infarct after left putaminal hemorrhage (*arrow*). **B** Pure-tone audiometry shows bilateral mild sensory hearing loss. **C** Speech audiometry shows large right–left differences. **D** Dichotic listening test reveals even greater right–left differences

- The dichotic listening test demonstrated that there was ipsilateral ear advantage in patients with left and/or right auditory cortex or auditory radiation lesions (Fig. 4).
- Environmental sounds were normally perceived in the right and left auditory cortex of auditory radiation lesions (1).
- Auditory evoked responses. Auditory brainstem responses (ABRs), middle-latency responses (MLR), and long-latency responses (LLRs) were normal in both ears.

These results revealed that auditory information processing for speech discrimination and auditory comprehension could be severely affected by lesions in the higher level of the auditory pathway.

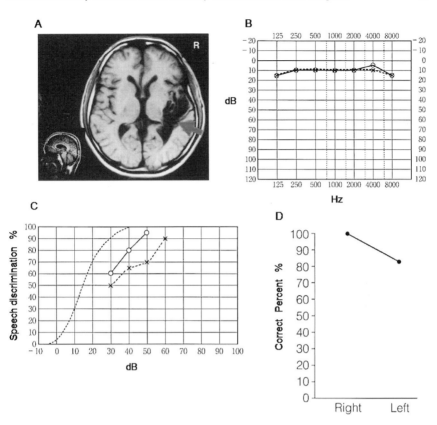

Fig. 2. A 37-year-old man with a lesion of the right superior temporal gyrus caused by hemorrhage due to an arteriovenous malformation. **A** Brain magnetic resonance imaging shows a large infarct after right temporal lobe hemorrhage (*arrow*). **B** Pure-tone audimetry shows normal hearing of both ears. **C** Speech audimetry shows small right–left differences. **D** Dichotic listening test reveals the left auditory neglect

Pure Word Deafness

Pure word deafness is defined as a selective deficit of auditory language comprehension and is distinguished from cortical auditory deficits by the absence of deficits in understanding music and environmental sounds (2–4). Lichtheim (1885) suggested that this syndrome was due to the isolation of Wernicke's area from auditory linguistic input following damage to the subcortex of the left temporal lobe. Liepmann and Storch (1902) supported this view in the light of autopsy studies, and more recently, Geschwind (1965) advocated a similar view. Thereafter, many cases labeled as pure word deafness have been reported with anatomical documentation of either unilateral left or bilateral cortical/subcortical damage to the temporal lobe. The number of cases that comply with the above definition of pure word deafness is, however, much smaller; and in only a few has the location of the lesion been precisely delineated (2–4).

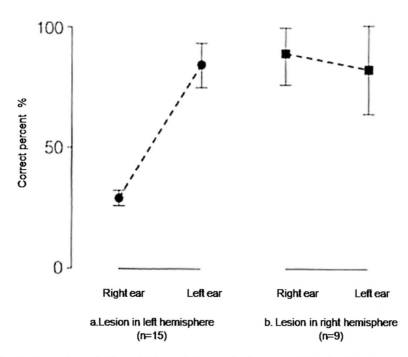

Fig. 3. Comparison of right and left ear differences in the monosyllable discrimination rate in (**a**) patients with a lesion of the left auditory cortex and radiation, and (**b**) patients (n = 9) with a lesion of the right auditory cortex and radiation

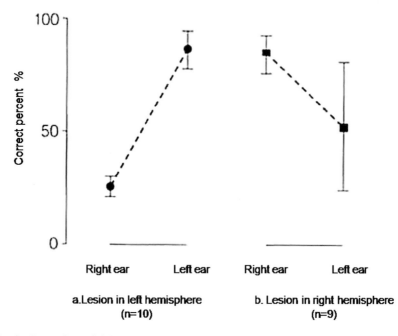

Fig. 4. Comparison of right and left ear differences in the dichotic listening test in (**a**) patients with a lesion of the left auditory cortex and radiation (n = 10), and (**b**) patients with a lesion of the right auditory cortex and radiation (n = 9)

References

1. Kaga K, Shindo M, Sugishita M (1987) Speech and sound recognition in an auditory pathway: vocalization vs. non-vocalization. Technical report. The Institute of Electronics, Information and Communication Engineers, Tokyo, pp 9–16
2. Metz-lutz MN, Dahl E (1984) Analysis of word comprehension in a case of pure word-deafness. Brain Lang 23:13–25
3. Okada S, Hanada M, Hattori H, et al (1963) A case of pure word-deafness (about the relation between auditory perception and recognition of speech-sound). Studia Phonologica1 4:58–65
4. Henschen SE (1917) Uber die Hörsphare. J Psychol Neurol 22:319–474

Unilateral Auditory Cortex Lesion and Middle-Latency Auditory-Evoked Magnetic Fields[1]

Introduction

The generators of auditory middle-latency responses (AMLRs) have been controversial in animal experiments (1, 2) and clinical studies (3–5). The critical issue is whether the auditory cortex contributes to the AMLR. The AMLR has been used for functional diagnoses in patients with auditory imperceptions, such as word deafness or auditory agnosia (4).

The conventional MLR, which is recorded from the patient's scalp, is a far-field recording of electric potential differences generated by neural currents. The signal is significantly affected by intervening tissues, such as the scalp, cranial bones, and cerebrospinal fluid. Also, multiple generators cannot be isolated in such recordings. In contrast, the magnetic field generated by the electric current in neurons is measured with magnetic encephalography (MEG). As the magnetic permeability of the intervening tissues is almost the same as that of air, the magnetic field can be measured on the surface of the scalp with little distortion. MEG is particularly effective in localizing signals from axons that are oriented perpendicular to the scalp, such as those in the cortex and its projections. Its precision in mapping such generators is enhanced by the fact that the field strength from these sources falls rapidly with distance (6, 7). Hence, MEG is suited to the precise localization of activity sources in the brain. As an indicator of auditory cortex function in MEG, the N1m is widely used for basic and clinical studies (8, 9). There have been only a few studies of the Pam of middle-latency auditory-evoked magnetic fields (MLAEFs), which are also localized in the auditory cortex (10–13); and no auditory cortex lesion study of the Pam of MLAEFs has been reported.

---

[1]This section of the chapter was excerpted from: Kaga K, Kurauchi T, Yumoto M, Uno A. Middle-latency auditory-evoked magnetic fields in patients with auditory cortex lesions. *Acta Otolaryngol* 124:376–380, 2004.

The aim of this study was to demonstrate the influence of unilateral auditory cortex lesions on the Pa of AMLRs and the Pam of MLAEFs using simultaneous recordings in patients with such lesions (Figs. 1–3).

Subject and Methods

A total of 15 controls participated in this study as well as 9 patients with left auditory cortex lesions who manifested sensory aphasia. They were all right-handed and had normal hearing. In all patients, the left primary and secondary auditory cortices had been damaged by cerebrovascular accidents. In addition, one patient with a right auditory cortex lesion was studied.

Middle-latency auditory magnetic fields were recorded in a magnetically shielded room using a 37-channel SQUID gradiometer (Magnes; Biomagnetic Technologies, San Diego, CA, USA), and AMLRs were recorded simultaneously for comparison. The patient was recumbent on a bed with his or her head fixed by a vacuum cushion. Auditory stimulation was provided by tone bursts (2000 Hz, 100.2 dB peSPL, rise/ fall time 0.1 ms, plateau 10 ms) that were delivered to one ear of the subject through a plastic tube. The stimulus rate was 2 Hz, with 3000 repetitions. The sensor array (144 mm diameter) was located as close as possible to the auditory cortex on the side opposite to the stimulated ear and was recorded by right or left ear stimulation separately. Simultaneously, AMLRs were recorded using surface electrodes placed at Cz (vertex), C3 (over the left temporal lobe), and C4 (over the right temporal lobe). The ground electrode was placed on the ear lobe of the stimulated ear. The recording bandwidth was 1–2000 Hz. The peak latency (milliseconds) and amplitude (root-mean square [r.m.s.] values in the case of the MLAEF) were measured.

Results

Simultaneous recordings of AMLB and MLAEFs of a normal subject are shown in Fig. 1. The dipoles of the MLAEFs were seen to be superimposed on the auditory cortex on MRI. Figure 2 shows MLAEFs and the dipole localization fitted to a brain MRI scan for a typical patient, a 64-year-old man. The MLAEF is absent from the left hemisphere but is present from the right hemisphere; the AMLRs are present in biolateral hemispheres. Figure 3 shows AMLRs and MLAEFs in the right auditory cortex lesion as well as the dipole localization fitted to the brain MRI scan for a typical patient, a 63-year-old man. The Pa of the AMLRs and MLAEFs was present from the left hemisphere in response to a right-ear stimulus. The Pam from the right hemisphere in response to a left stimulus was absent, but the Pam from the left hemisphere was present in response to a right-ear stimulus; the Pa of the AMLR was present from both hemispheres.

The average latency and amplitude of the Pa in the AMLRs and the Pam in the MLAEFs from the right and left hemispheres are shown in Fig. 4. There is no

a.

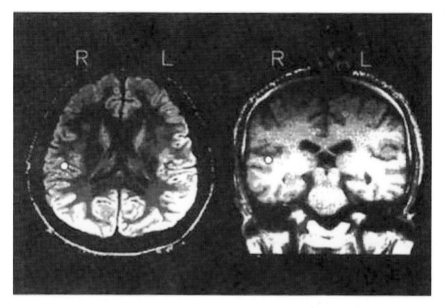

b.

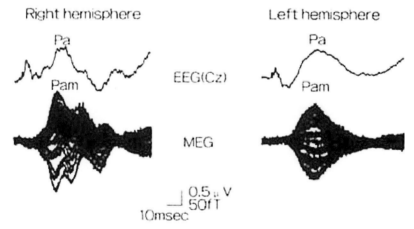

Fig. 1. **a** Superimposition of the dipole (ECD) on the auditory cortex of the brain magnetic resonance (MRI) scan. A *white circle* indicates the site of the ECD. **b** Typical simultaneous recordings
of auditory middle-latency responses (AMLRs) and middle-latency auditory-evoked magnetic
fields (MLAEFs) in a normal subject, a 25-year-old man. Right- and left-hemisphere recordings
were made with contralateral stimulation. *EEG*, electroencephalography; *MEG*, magnetic
encephalography

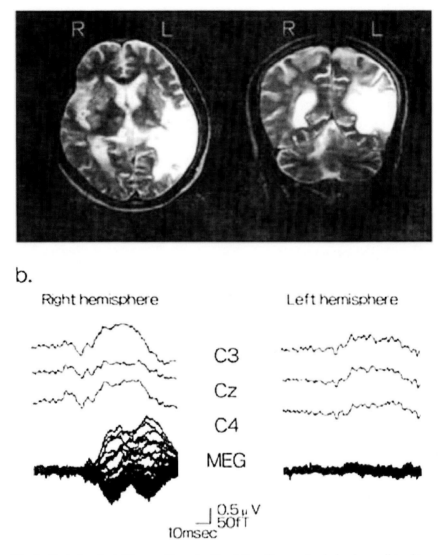

Fig. 2. Typical patient (64-year-old man) with a left auditory cortex lesion in a unilateral tem-poroparietal infarction. **a** Brain MRI scans. AMLRs and MLAEFs are shown. **b** The MLAEF is absent from the left hemisphere but is present in the right hemisphere. However, the AMLRs are present from the bilateral hemispheres

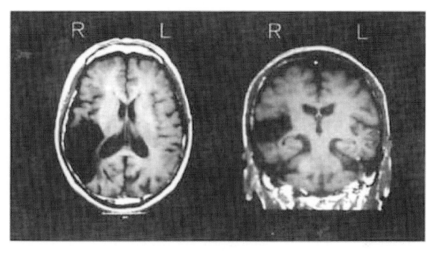

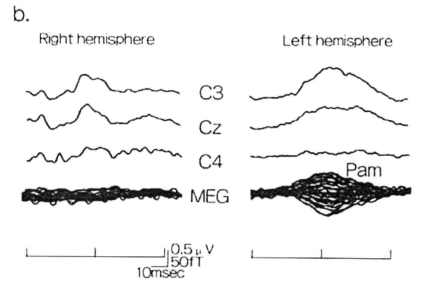

Fig. 3. Typical patient (63-year-old man) with a right auditory cortex lesion in a unilateral temporoparietal infarction. **a** Brain MRI scans. **b** AMLRs and MLAEFs are shown. The MLAEF is absent from the right hemisphere, but the AMRL is present from both hemispheres

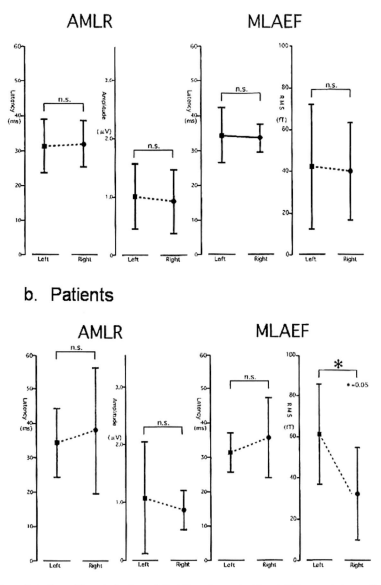

Fig. 4. **a** Data from 15 controls showed that there is no significant difference between the left and right hemispheres (right-ear and left-ear stimulation) in terms of the latency or amplitude of the AMLR or MLAEFs. **b** In nine patients with left-hemisphere lesions, the MLAEF amplitude is significantly reduced for right-ear stimulation

significant difference in the latency or amplitude of the Pa from the right and left hemispheres in the AMLRs. However, there is a significant difference in the r.m.s. amplitude of the Pam from the right and left hemispheres on MEG; there was no significant left–right difference in Pam latency.

Dipole locations of equivalent current dipoles (ECDs) with relative coefficients >0.98 were calculated. For the right hemisphere, eight of nine patients had coefficients >0.98; only one of nine patients had no such correlation for the left hemisphere. Statistically, for the right hemisphere there was no difference between normal subjects and patients (Fig. 4). A comparison between the left and right hemispheres among the patients, using paired t-tests, showed a significant difference in amplitude ($P < 0.05$) in eight patients. The other patient, whose relative coefficient was >0.98, did not show significant differences between the right and left hemispheres (Fig. 2).

Comment

Compared to the Pa component of the AMLR, the Pam of the MLAEF is substantially more sensitive to the activity of the auditory cortex ipsilateral to the magnetic sensor. The primary generator of the Pam in MLAEFs has been demonstrated to be the auditory cortex. However, the Pa of AMLRs is evoked only partly from the auditory cortex because it is evoked even in patients with unilateral auditory cortex lesions.

References

1. Kraus N, Ozdamar O, Hier D, et al (1982) Auditory middle latency responses (MLRs) in patients with cortical lesions. Electroencephalogr Clin Neurophysiol 54:275–287
2. Woods DL, Clayworth CC, Knight RT, et al (1987) Generators of middle- and long-latency auditory evoked potentials; implications from studies of patients with bitemporal lesions. Electroencephalogr Clin Neurophysiol 68:132–148
3. Ibanez V, Deiber MP, Fisher C (1989) Middle latency auditory evoked potentials in cortical lesions: criteria of interhemispheric asymmetry. Arch Neurol 46:1325–1332
4. Panev C, Lütkenhöner B, Hoke M, et al (1986) Comparison between simultaneously recorded auditory-evoked magnetic fields and potentials elicited by ipsilateral, contralateral and binaural tone burst stimulation. Auditory 25:54–61
5. Pelizzone M, Hari R, Makela JP, et al (1987) Cortical origin of middle-latency auditory evoked responses in man. Neurosci Lett 82:303–307
6. Makela JP, Hamalainen M, Hari R, et al (1994) Whole-head mapping of middle-latency auditory evoked magnetic fields. Electroencephalogr Clin Neurophysiol 92:414–421
7. Yoshiura T, Ueno S, Iamina K, et al (1994) Effects of stimulation side on human middle latency auditory evoked magnetic fields. Neurosci Lett 172:159–162
8. Kuriki S, Nogai T, Hirasta Y (1995) Cortical sources of middle latency responses of auditory evoked magnetic field. Hear Res 92:47–51

9. Kaga K, Kurauchi T, Yumoto M, et al (2004) Middle-latency auditory-evoked magnetic fields in patients with auditory cortex lesions. Acta Otolaryngol 124:376–380

10. Pelizzone M, Hari R, Makela JP, et al (1987) Cortical origin of middle-latency auditory evoked responses in man. Neurosci Lett 82:303–307

11. Makela JP, Hamalainen M, Hari R, et al (1994) Whole-head mapping of middle-latency auditory evoked magnetic fields. Electroencephalogr Clin Neurophysiol 92:414–421

12. Yoshiura T, Ueno S, Iramina K, et al (1994) Effects of stimulation side on human middle latency auditory evoked magnetic fields. Neurosci Lett 172:159–162

13. Kuriki S, Nogai T, Hirata Y (1995) Cortical sources of middle latency responses of auditory evoked magnetic field. Hear Res 92:47–51

7
Bilateral Auditory Cortex and/or Auditory Radiation Lesion and Perception

[1]Severe auditory deficit due to bilateral lesions of the primary auditory cortex or auditory radiation is rare. This serious hearing problem is called "auditory agnosia" or "cortical deafness." Most studies on humans are single or double case reports (1–6) and have led us to question whether bilateral lesions in the human primary auditory cortex can cause complete deafness. However, in animal experiments, Neff et al. (7) noted that bilateral ablation of the primary auditory cortex does not cause permanent deafness, with preservation of pure-tone thresholds.

Since the introduction of computed tomography (CT), magnetic resonance imaging (MRI), and auditory brainstem responses (ABRs) for clinical use, we have seen more than 10 patients who lost auditory cortices and/or radiations bilaterally after cerebrovascular accidents (CVAs). Despite these bilateral lesions, the patients have not lost all hearing; rather, their hearing is somewhat disturbed, with confusion in regard to what they can or cannot hear. We focused specifically on their central auditory processing using a battery of perceptional tests for hearing.

Case Reports

Case 1

A 24-year-old woman had moyamoya disease. The lesion was shown by MRI to be located bilaterally in the auditory cortex and radiation (Fig. 1). Pure-tone audiometry showed a normal hearing threshold two years after onset and ABRs and K complex on EEG were well elicited (Fig. 1). Monosyllable tests of both ears (with scores of 2%) and the Token test (score of 22%) indicated severe impairment.

---

[1]This section of the chapter was excerpted from: Kaga K, Shindo M, Tanaka Y. Central auditory information processing in patients with bilateral auditory cortex lesions. *Acta Otolaryngol Suppl* (*Stockh*) 532:77–82, 1997.

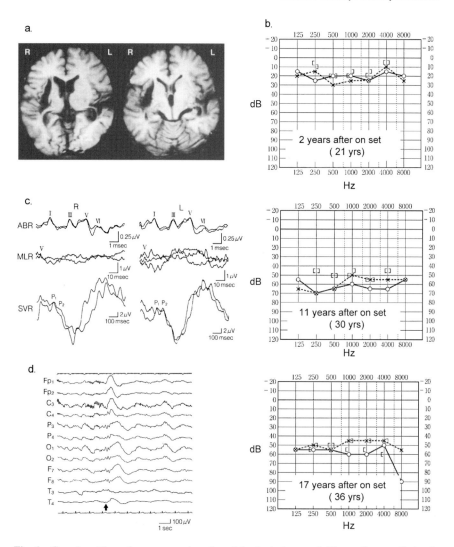

Fig. 1. Case 1. **a** Magnetic resonance imaging of the brain in case 1. The auditory radiation in the right hemisphere is lesioned; and the auditory cortex and radiation in the left hemisphere are damaged. **b** Pure-tone audiometry shows progressive sensory neural hearing loss. **c** There are normal auditory brainstem responses (ABRs) and slow vertex responses (SVRs) but absent middle latency responses (MLRs) in both ears. **d** Electroencephalography (EEG) shows that K complexes to a sound stimulus are recorded from all leads (**d**, *arrow*)

In the lip reading tests, the score for lip reading plus listening for words was 48%, which was markedly better than that for lip reading alone (12%) or listening alone (0%). For short sentences, the score for lip reading plus listening (20%) was a little better than that for lip reading alone (0%) or listening alone (10%).

Case 2

A 53-year-old woman had subarachnoid hemorrhage. The lesion was located in the left auditory radiation and the right auditory cortex (Fig. 2). Pure-tone audiometry showed apparently mild sensory hearing deficit, but the ABR was normal. The monosyllable test scores in other ears was 0%. On the other hand, the Token test score was 57%. The score for lip reading plus listening for words was 68%, which was better than that for lip reading alone (40%) or listening alone (24%). For short sentences, the score for lip reading plus listening (80%) was markedly better than that for lip reading alone (10%) or listening alone (10%).

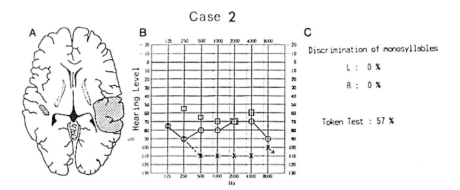

Fig. 2. Case 2. **A** Lesion sites demonstrated by computed tomography (CT). **B** Audiogram showed mild threshold elevation in spite of normal ABRs. **C** Discrimination of 53 Japanese nonsense monosyllables. *L*, left ear; *R*, right ear. Token test was 57%

Case 3

A 65-year-old man had a cerebral infarction with the bilateral lesion located in the auditory cortex (Fig. 3). Pure-tone audiometry showed near-normal hearing. The monosyllable test scores were only 8% in the right ear and 15% in the left. On the other hand, the Token test score was 62%. The score for lip reading plus listening for words was 36%, which was better than that for lip reading alone (10%) or listening alone (24%). For short sentences, the score for lip reading plus listening (20%) was a little better than that for lip reading alone (0%) or listening alone (0%).

Case **3**

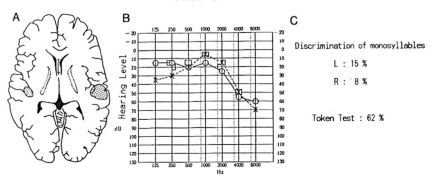

Fig. 3. Case 3. **A** Lesion sites demonstrated by CT. **B** Audiogram. **C** Discrimination of 53 Japanese nonsense monosyllables. Token test was 62%

Table 1. Patient characteristics

Case	Sex	Onset (year)	Age (years)	Etiology	Lesions	Remarks
1	F	1979	24	Cerebral bleeding	Lt. auditory radiation Rt. auditory cortex	Moyamoya disease
2	F	1979	53	Cerebral bleeding	Bilat. auditory cortex	
3	M	1981	65	Cerebral bleeding	Bilat. auditory cortex	
4	M	1984	75	Cerebral bleeding	Bilat. auditory cortex	
5	M	1984	50	Cerebral bleeding	Bilat. auditory cortex	
6	M	1984	25	Cerebral bleeding	Bilat. auditory cortex	Leukemia
7	M	1985	64	Cerebral bleeding	Bilat. auditory cortex	
8	M	1985	22	Cerebral bleeding	Bilat. auditory cortex	Leukemia
9	F	1991	48	Cerebral bleeding	Bilat. auditory cortex	
10	M	1975	Died in 1989	Cerebral bleeding	Bilat. auditory cortex	Autopsy

Audiological Results

The profiles of the 10 patients participating in this study are shown in Table 1. All patients had bilateral lesions in the auditory cortex and/or auditory radiation.

- *Pure-tone audiometry* revealed a normal, mild, or moderate range of thresholds in each patient. No patients had profound hearing loss.
- *Auditory brainstem responses* appeared normal at 85 dB HL with the low threshold around 20–30 dB nHL. Thus, peripheral hearing loss was ruled out in all patients.
- *Speech discrimination test for auditory perception.* A total of 53 nonsense monosyllables (e.g., ex, pa, mi, tsu) were selected among 100 monosyllables from the Japanese language. The sounds were tape-recorded and delivered to each ear separately through headphones at an intensity of 50 dB above the subjective threshold. Each patient was asked to identify each monosyllable orally or

in writing. The following results were obtained for normal-hearing subjects: 53 nonsense monosyllables were identified correctly at a percentage of 84% ± 7%. No right–left ear differences were found (average age 29.5 years; $n = 20$). All of the patients showed almost 0% correct identification in the nonsense monosyllable perception test.

- *Environmental sound perception test.* A total of 24 environmental sounds were classified into five categories: 1) human voice; 2) animal and bird calls; 3) musical instruments; 4) natural noises; and 5) artificial noises (Fig. 4). The

Test Sounds		Response (n=10)	
		Oral Answer	Picture Matching
a. Human	1. Man's Voice	●●	●●●●
	2. Woman's Voice		●●
	3. Song	●●	●●●●●
	4. Baby's Cry	●	●●●●●●●●●●
	5. Laugh		●●●●
	6. English		●●●●
b. Animal	1. Cat		●●●●●●●
and Bird	2. Dog	●	●●●●●
	3. Cow	●	●●●●●●
	4. Horse		●
	5. Crow		●●●●●
	6. Cock		●●●●
c. Instrument	1. Drum	●●●●●	●●●●●●●●
	2. Trumpet	●	●●●●●
	3. Clock	●	●●●●●
	4. Telephone	●	●●●●●●●
d. Nature	1. Wind	●	●●●●●
	2. Wave		●●●
	3. Stream		●
e. Noise	1. Train	●●	●●●●●●
	2. Car		●
	3. Gun		●●●●●
	4. Saw	●	●●●●
	5. Foot Steps		●●●●●

Fig. 4. Summary of the environmental sound perception test. Each *black circle* indicates a patient who can correctly identify each item of the test sounds. Oral answers and picture matching are compared

first test consists of two steps. The first step is just to listen and identify each sound orally or in writing. The second step was a picture-matching test. The sound source was chosen from a set of four pictures. With the environmental sounds, the percentage of correct responses in the oral report and picture matching was 100% (average age 35 years; $n = 20$). For oral identification of environmental sounds, most patients could not answer each item correctly except for drum sounds. With picture matching, however, more than half of the patients could identify several items correctly. Those items were a baby crying, cat, cow, drum, trumpet, clock, telephone, wind, train, gun, and footsteps (Fig. 4).

- *Token test for auditory comprehension.* This test, devised by Renzi and Vignolo (8), was used to determine the degree of impairment of auditory comprehension. Each patient was tested using oral speech sounds with the examiner's mouth concealed from the patient's view. For the Token tests, the percentage of correct responses was 98% ± 3% (average age 44.9 years; $n = 54$). All of the patients scored less than 50% percent in the Token test.

Comment

Our study reveals that auditory information processing for loudness of pure tones and monosyllable discrimination, environment sound perception, and auditory comprehension is commonly, but differently, affected by bilateral lesions in the auditory cortex or auditory radiation. The differences are probably due to differences in the size of the lesions.

Discrimination of nonsense monosyllables was severely impaired, and auditory comprehension (determined by the Token test) was moderately or severely impaired. For a comparison, in our study on 70-year-old people, pure-tone audiometry showed mild elevation in the hearing threshold, but nonsense monosyllable speech audiometry revealed slight impairment of a maximum discrimination score of 10%–30%. The Token test showed a normal or subnormal range of auditory comprehension, around 90%. This characteristic of hearing in elderly people means that presbycusis is caused mostly by sensory neural hearing loss at the cochlea, not by abnormal central auditory processing at the auditory cortex.

However, the perception of environmental sounds in patients with bilateral auditory cortex and radiation lesions was partially preserved (3, 6). The common features of these sounds are impulsive and repetitive. However, most of the patients could not identify the sounds of a horse, a stream, or a car (Fig. 1). This may be due to the weak distinctive features of these noises. It is important to note that environmental sounds were identified by these patients when picture matching was added.

The present study also demonstrates that for three representative patients auditory comprehension improved when lip reading was combined with listening, compared with lip reading alone or listening alone. In the case of simple conversation, they could understand family members or acquaintances by reading their lips. For more complicated conversation however, they relied on written communication. In this study, the lip-reading-only scores for these patients were lower than those for controls in tests for both words and short sentences. The scores for lip reading combined with listening, however, were better than those for lip reading only in tests for both words and short sentences. Auerbach et al. (4) reported that auditory comprehension could be improved in patients with pure word deafness by combining listening with lip reading. Lip reading helps in the auditory perception of speech, an ability that appears to be preserved even in patients with auditory agnosia. It is clear that patients with auditory agnosia without aphasia can use lip reading to improve their comprehension of speech (9).

It remains to be fully understood why residual hearing is usually maintained in our patients. There are at least two possibilities to explain central auditory information processing after bilateral lesions of the auditory cortex or radiation. One is the possibility of a contribution of nonspecific auditory pathways to perceive particular environmental sounds and to improve lip reading ability with the help of listening although the cortical center of nonspecific auditory pathways is unknown. Finally, it is important for understanding the human auditory system to illuminate central auditory processing after loss of the bilateral auditory cortex, such as was described here.

References

1. Jerger J, Weikers NJ, Sharbrough III FW, et al (1969) Bilateral lesions of the temporal lobe: a case study. Acta Otolaryngol (Stockh) Suppl 258:1–51
2. Oppenheimer DR, Newcombe F (1978) Clinical and anatomic findings in a case of auditory agnosia. Arch Neurol 35:712–719
3. Shindo M, Kaga K, Tanaka Y (1981) Auditory agnosia following bilateral temporal bone lesion: report of a case. Brain Nerve (Tokyo) 33:139–147
4. Auerbach SH, Allard T, Naeser M, et al (1982) Pure word deafness: an analysis of a case with bilateral lesions and a defect at the prephonemic level. Brain 105:271–300
5. Woods DL, Knight RT, Neville HJ (1984) Bitemporal lesions dissociate auditory evoked potentials and perception. Electroencephalogr Clin Neurophysiol 57:208–220
6. Tanaka Y, Kamo T, Yoshida M, et al (1991) Clinical and anatomical findings. Brain 114:2385–2401
7. Neff WD, Diamond IT, Casseday JH (1975) Behavioral studies of auditory discrimination: central nervous system. In: Keidel WD, Neff WD (eds) Handbook of sensory physiology. Vol 5. Part 2. Springer, Berlin, pp 307–400
8. De Renzi E, Vignolo LA (1962) A sensitive test to detect receptive disturbances in aphasics. Brain 85:665–678
9. Shindo M, Kaga K, Tanaka Y (1991) Speech discrimination and lip reading in patients with word deafness or auditory agnosia. Brain Lang 40:153–161

Neuropathology of Auditory Agnosia Following Bilateral Temporal Lobe Lesions[2]

The brain pathology of auditory agnosia or cortical deafness has been reported rarely. Moreover, most of that reported did not contain modern audiological data and brain MRI. We illustrate audiological data and pathological findings of a particular case.

Case Report

Our patient was first diagnosed with auditory agnosia following his second CVA in 1975 when he was 37 years old (Fig. 1). Comprehensive follow-up examinations of auditory function were conducted periodically until his sudden death 15 years later. His brain was studied postmortem for neuropathology. Initial pure-tone audiometry revealed moderate sensorineural hearing loss in the right ear and mild sensorineural hearing loss in the left ear. However, repeated pure-tone audiometry revealed that

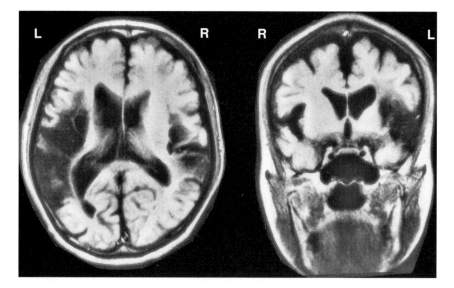

Fig. 1. Brain computed tomography shows a large infarct in the left hemisphere and a small infarct in the right hemisphere including the auditory cortex. **a** Horizontal slice. **b** Coronal slice

[2]This section of the chapter was excerpted from: Kaga K, Shindo M, Tanaka Y, Haebara H. Neuropathology of auditory agnosia following bilateral temporal lobe lesions: a case study. *Acta Otolaryngol* 120:259–262, 2000.

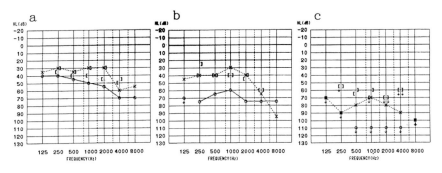

Fig. 2. Chronological changes of the audiogram. **a** Four years after onset (40 years old). **b** Nine years after onset (45 years old). **c** One year before death (49 years old)

bilaterally the thresholds became progressively poorer over time (Fig. 2). Speech audiometry of both ears consistently revealed that the patient was unable to discriminate any monosyllabic words (i.e., speech intelligibility scores were 0% bilaterally). In general, speech and hearing tests demonstrated that he could not comprehend spoken words but could comprehend written commands and gestures. Postmortem neuropathological study of the left hemispheres revealed a total defect (Fig. 3) and neuronal loss of the superior temporal gyrus, including Heschl's gyrus, and total gliosis of the medial geniculate body (Fig. 4a). In the right hemisphere, examination revealed subcortical necrosis, gliosis in the center of the superior temporal gyrus, and partial gliosis of the medial geniculate body (Fig. 4b). The pathology examination supported the clinical results in which the patient's imperception of speech sounds, music, and environmental sounds could be caused by progressive degeneration of the bilateral medial geniculate body.

Comment

In the previous literature of autopsied cases with bilateral audiometry cortex lesions, pure-tone thresholds have been categorized as having either mild or severe elevation. However, thresholds varied across studies. For example, some cases demonstrated mild threshold elevation (1–3), whereas others showed thresholds that were seriously elevated (4, 5). The audiograms were not completed during the clinical course for these patients across cases or studies. Part of the problem with previous studies is that they completed only one audiogram, whereas in our case, pure-tone audiometry was completed repeatedly during the clinical course, and progressive threshold elevation was observed. At an early stage after the onset of our patient's disease, he showed mild threshold elevation. Later examinations revealed that the threshold had become progressively poorer and finally reached severe to profound levels 1 year before his death.

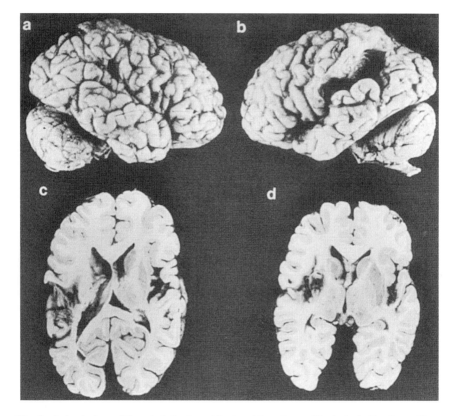

Fig. 3. Lateral view of the whole brain and horizontal sections of brain including the auditory cortex. **a** Right hemisphere. A small infarct is observed in the upper part of the Sylvian fissure. **b** Left hemisphere. Extensive infarction is observed in Broca's areas; the first was observed in Broca's area, the first temporal gyrus, and the supramarginal gyrus. **c** This section shows a large infarct in the left hemisphere. **d** In this section, bilateral infarction of the auditory cortex is observed, but the right infarct is smaller than the left infarct

The pathology examination for our patient showed the disappearance and degeneration of neuronal cells in the medial geniculate body, as was seen in other reported cases (2–7). The pathophysiology was thought to be due to retrograde degeneration of auditory radiations or neuronal fibers of the medial geniculate body (8). Yamada and Kaga (9) reported that changes in the middle latency response and the retrograde degeneration occur slowly in cats with bilateral auditory cortex ablation. Hirano (5) reported that profound hearing loss was caused by total degeneration of the medial geniculate body. The current pathology examination supports the clinical results indicating that the patient's imperception of speech sounds, music, and environmental sounds could be caused by progressive degeneration of the bilateral medial geniculate body.

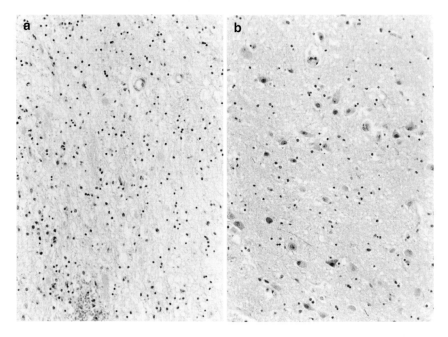

Fig. 4. Histology of the medial geniculate body. **a** Neuronal cells of the left medial geniculate body have been completely replaced by glial cells. **b** Neuronal cells of the right medial geniculate body have been partially replaced by glial cells. There is partial neuronal cell preservation. (H&E, ×200)

In conclusion, degeneration of the medial geniculate body may have occurred as a result of retrograde degeneration due to bilateral auditory cortex lesions.

References

1. Leicesserf J (1980) Central deafness and subcortical motor aphasia. Brain Lang 10:224–242
2. Lhermitte F, Chain F, Escouroller R, et al (1971) [Study of auditory perception disorders in bilateral temporal lesions. (3 case studies 2 of which are anatomoclinical).] Rev Neurol (Paris) 124:329–351
3. Kaga K, Shindo M, Tanaka Y (1997) Central auditory information processing in patients with bilateral auditory cortex lesions. Acta Otolaryngol (Stockh) 532:S77–S82
4. Bahls FH, Chatrial GE, Mesher RA, et al (1988) A case of persistent cortical deafness: clinical neurophysiologic, and neuropathologic observations. Neurology 38:1490–1493
5. Hirano M (1976) Autopsy findings of a case with so-called cortical deafness. Clin Neurol Jpn 16:962–966
6. Clark WE, Le G, Russell WR (1938) Cortical deafness without aphasia. Brain 61:375–383
7. Oppenheimer DR (1978) Clinical and anatomic findings in a case of auditory agnosia. Arch Neurol 35:712–719

8. Csilik B, Toth L (1987) Degeneration, axonal. In: Adelman G (ed) Encyclopedia of neuroscience. Vol 1. Birskhauser, Boston, pp 304–306
9. Yamada K, Kaga K (1995) Long-term changes in middle latency response and the evidence of retrograde degeneration in the media geniculate body after auditory cortical ablation in cats. Audiol Jpn 36:725–726

Preservation of the Auditory Cortex and Bilateral Lesions Confined to the Auditory Radiation: MEG and PET Studies of a Patient with Auditory Agnosia[3]

There are two parallel auditory systems in the brain. The most important system is the primary auditory pathway, which conveys neural signals of speech, music, and environmental sounds from the cochlea through the cochlear nerve, brainstem auditory pathway, and medial geniculate, to the auditory radiation and auditory cortex. The other system is the nonspecific auditory pathway, which conveys neural signals from the cochlea through the pontine and thalamic reticular formation or the medical geniculate body to the cerebral cortex.

The aim of this study was to investigate whether function is absent or present in the auditory cortex of a patient with auditory agnosia due to bilateral lesions of auditory radiations but a preserved auditory cortex. The investigation was conducted using magnetic encephalography (MEG), auditory evoked responses, and position emission tomography (PET). Many MEG studies of auditory cortex function have been reported in normal subjects, but studies of patients with auditory cortex lesions are rarely reported; moreover, there have been no studies reported of bilateral auditory radiation lesions with preservation of the auditory cortex.

Case Report

A patient experienced left mild temporal hemiplegia because of right putaminal hemorrhage at the age of 43. Thereafter, he recovered completely but hypertension persisted. When he was 53 years old, he went into a coma due to left putaminal hemorrhage. After he recovered from the coma, he manifested mild right hemiplegia and hearing problems. The hemiplegia resolved except for some residual weakness, but the auditory problems persisted. He found that he could not discriminate any speech, music, or environmental sounds even though he could hear them. Brain CT and MRI demonstrated localized small lesions in only the bilateral auditory radiation (Fig. 1). Pure-tone audiometry revealed bilateral mild hearing loss (Fig. 2).

---

[3]This section of the chapter was excerpted from: Kaga K, Kurauchi T, Nakamura M, et al. Magnetoencephalography and positron emission tomography studies of patients with auditory agnosia caused by bilateral lesions confined to the auditory radiations. *Acta Otolaryngol* 125:1351–1355, 2005.

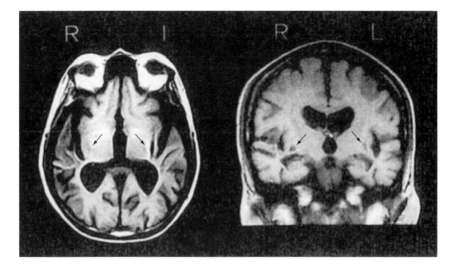

Fig. 1. Magnetic resonance imaging scan of the patient's brain. In both hemispheres, auditory radiations are damaged by small areas of infarction (*arrows*)

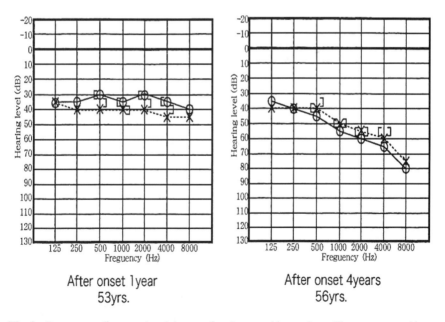

Fig. 2. Pure-tone audiograms 1 and 4 years after the second hemorrhage. The tests reported here were performed at the time of the second audiogram

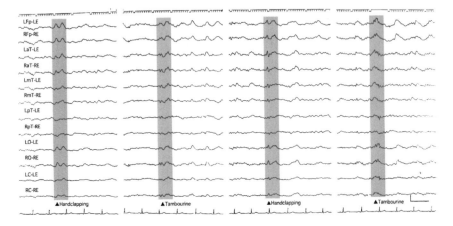

Fig. 3. Electroencephalography recording. The K complex appeared in response to sounds (*shadow areas*)

Auditory evoked potential studies demonstrated normal electrocochleography (EcochG), ABRs and middle-latency response (MLR). The K complex to sound stimuli was clearly recorded on electroencephalography (EEG) (Fig. 3). Neuropsychological tests demonstrated that he could not discriminate any speech, music, or environmental sounds but that he had no aphasia. He was diagnosed as having auditory agnosia due to bilateral lesions confined to the auditory radiation, with preservation and isolation of the auditory cortex bilaterally. Subsequently, his pure-tone threshold worsened in the higher frequencies (Fig. 2).

Magnetic encephalography and auditory evoked response studies were conducted 4 years later, at the time of the second audiogram (seen in Fig. 2). They demonstrated that the middle-latency auditory magnetic fields (MLAEFs) and auditory middle-latency responses (AMLRs) were absent with a very small Pa of the AMLRs (Fig. 4). On the other hand, a positron emission tomography (PET) study demonstrated increased blood flow in the bilateral auditory cortex in response to clicks and Japanese monosyllable verbal stimuli (Japanese monosyllables generally correspond to consonant-vowel sounds in English). Cerebral blood flow increased by at least 10% over the resting baseline in areas of the auditory cortex, especially with verbal stimuli, but did not reach the 20% increases that are typical in normal subjects (Fig. 5).

Comment

Because the auditory cortex was not damaged in this patient, our aim was to investigate with objective measures whether the auditory cortex could respond to auditory stimuli.

There are two auditory pathways in the brain (1–3). The most important one is the specific auditory pathway for auditory perception, and the other is the nonspecific

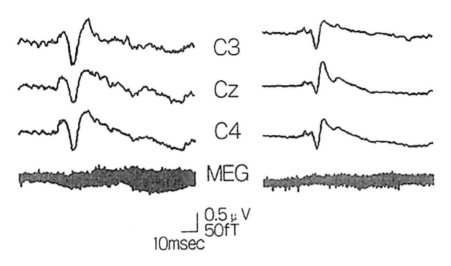

Fig. 4. Simultaneous recordings of the patient's auditory middle-latency responses (AMLRs) and middle-latency auditory magnetic fields (MLAEFs). Pam in the MLAEFs is absent in both hemispheres, but a very small Pa is present in the AMLRs of both hemispheres. *MEG*, magnetic encephalography

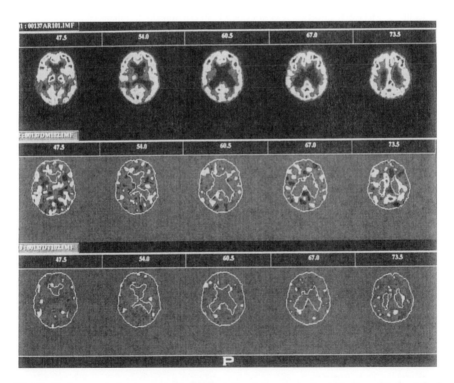

Fig. 5. Positron emission tomography (PET) study of changes in the patient's regional cerebral blood flow (rCBF) in response to clicks and verbal stimuli (100 monosyllables). *Top row*, averaged CBF images at rest; *middle row*, subtraction images of the CBF responding to clicks; *bottom row*, subtraction images of the CBF responding to verbal stimuli. Images are processed to show areas of 10% and 20% increase over the baseline blood flow. Some areas show a 10% increase for verbal stimuli and smaller areas activated by clicks. There are no areas with a 20% increase (as would be expected in normal individuals)

auditory pathway involved in arousal (2, 3). Although our patient's specific auditory pathway was damaged at the subcortical level of auditory radiation, the nonspecific auditory pathway was preserved. The PET study demonstrated increased blood flow in the auditory cortex at a level of 10% (approximately half of normal) in response to auditory stimuli. However, the absence of MLAEFs and AMLRs indicated impaired function of the specific auditory pathway because of the bilateral lesions of the auditory radiation (4–6). In patients with auditory cortex lesions, MLAEFs and AMLRs have been reported to be absent (6). However, it is significant that the patient could hear but could not discriminate most speech, music, or environmental sounds. This discrepancy is thought to be due to loss of the specific auditory pathway and preservation of the nonspecific auditory pathway. In this case, it was speculated that the auditory cortex received projections not only from the specific auditory pathway but also from the non-auditory-specific pathways in the cerebral hemispheres.

References

1. Rauschecker JP, Tian B (2000) Mechanisms and streams for processing of "what" and "where" in auditory cortex. Proc Natl Acad Sci USA 97:11800–11806
2. Kraus N, McGee T, Littsman T, et al (1992) Reticular formation influences on primary and non-primary auditory pathways as reflected by the middle latency response. Brain Res 587:186–194
3. Woods DL, Clayworth CC, Knight RT, et al (1987) Generators of middle- and long-latency auditory evoked potentials: implications from studies of patients with bitemporal lesions. Electroencephalogr Clin Neurophysiol 68:132–148
4. Pantev C, Hoke M, Lehnertz K, Lütkenhöner B (1989) Neuromagnetic evidence of an amplitopic organization of the human auditory cortex. Electroencephalogr Clin Neurophysiol 72:225–231
5. Pelizzone M, Hari R Mäkelä JP, et al (1987) Cortical origin of middle-latency auditory evoked responses in man. Neurosci Lett 92:414–421
6. Kaga K, Kurauchi T, Yumoto M, et al (2004) Middle-latency auditory evoked magnetic fields in patients with auditory cortex lesions. Acta Otolaryngol 124:376–380

Auditory Agnosia Due to Front Temporal Dementia[4]

After CVAs in adult patients, cortical deafness is caused by bilateral lesions of the auditory cortex or its radiations, whereas cortical anarthria or dysarthria is caused by lesions of Broca's area or corticobasilar lesions in the left hemisphere (1–3).

Generally, other than young children after herpes encephalitis, patients with cortical deafness do not present with articulation disorders (4, 5). Moreover, cortical

---

[4]This section of the chapter was excerpted from: Kaga K, Nakamura M, Takayama Y, Momose H. A case of cortical deafness and anarthria. *Acta Otolaryngol* 124:202–205, 2004.

anarthria or dysarthria is not ordinarily complicated by auditory problems. We report an unusual case manifesting as progressive cortical deafness and cortical anarthria simultaneously because of front temporal dementia, a degenerative disease.

Case Report

A woman born in 1929 grew up in Tokyo and graduated from high school. After she married, she worked at the accounting section in a small company. In 1999, she noticed hearing problems when using the telephone and an articulation disorder, which worsened rapidly over 2 years. She was referred to our university hospital in Tokyo for further examination of these problems.

Neurologically, except for the hearing and articulation problems, she exhibited no dysfunction of the motor or sensory system. Her speech and hearing had deteriorated to the point that she could not communicate orally, although she could communicate with family members and others by exchanging written messages. The Japanese system of writing involves *kanji*, Chinese characters, each of which has a meaning, plus *kana*, a phonetic system in which each symbol represents a syllable. Kana are used for such things as a suffixes for verbs and adjectives and for Japanese or foreign words that cannot be represented by kanji. This patient had no deficit in reading or writing kanji or kana.

Examinations

Audiological Tests

Pure-tone and speech audiometry demonstrated mildly elevated thresholds in the low and middle frequencies, but her maximum speech discrimination was 25% for the right ear and 20% for the left ear—far worse than the pure-tone thresholds would predict (Fig. 1).

Objective Audiometry

Distortion-product otoacoustic emissions (DPOAEs) were normal in both ears. ABRs demonstrated normal wave configuration at 90 dB and a normal threshold of 20 dB (Fig. 2). MLRs had normal wave configuration bilaterally. There was a difference between the right and left ears in the amplitude of NaPaNb, but this difference has no apparent clinical significance. The long-latency response (LLR) was normal with a slight, clinically insignificant right–left difference in N1P1N2.

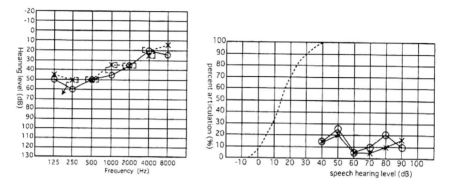

Fig. 1. Pure-tone audiometry. Thresholds are somewhat elevated for low and middle frequencies. Speech discrimination was no more than 25% at any sensation level

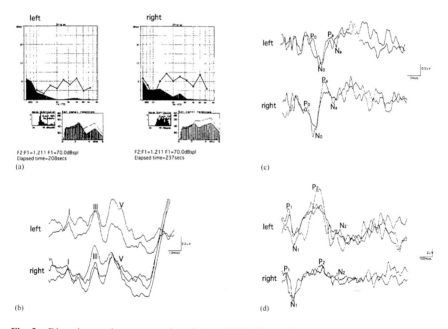

Fig. 2. Distortion-product otoacoustic emissions (DPOAEs), auditory brainstem responses (ABRs), middle-latency (MLR) and long-latency (LLR) responses are normal. The MLRs and LLRs have left–right differences of no known clinical significance but show all wave components bilaterally

Articulation Test and Sound Spectrography

An articulation test revealed marked abnormality for articulating words (3/50 correct) and sentences (0/10 correct) as well as for articulating vowels and consonants. Attempts to speak resulted in utterances of repetitive sounds, whose spectra demonstrated only F0 and F1.

Higher Brain Function Tests

- *Aphasia test*—Writing and reading skills were well preserved, but language skills that require hearing and speaking ability were markedly damaged.
- *Auditory perception test* (Token test)—This test for auditory comprehension (6) demonstrated a complete loss of auditory perception.
- *Environmental sound perception test* (2)—This test, which was developed by the authors using 24 sound materials, showed almost no responses: 0/24 in open-set testing and 4/24 with closed-set picture pointing.

Imaging Studies

- *MRI* (Fig. 3)—Brain MRI demonstrated atrophic changes of the primary auditory cortex, secondary auditory cortex, and motor cortex around the Sylvian fissures in both hemispheres.
- *PET studies based on glucose uptake* (Fig. 4)—Positron emission tomography of the local cerebral glucose metabolic rate was performed, with the patient given an injection of ^{18}F-2-fluoro-2-deoxy-D-glucose (FDG). There was decreased activity bilaterally in the auditory cortices, Broca's area, and Wernicke's area. Moreover, a slight or moderate decrease in glucose uptake was detected in the

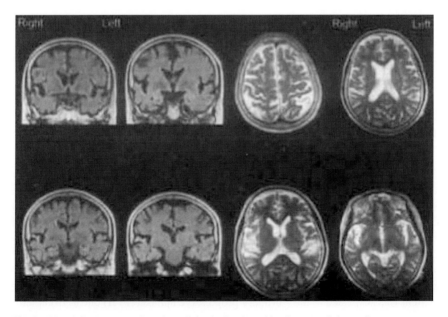

Fig. 3. Magnetic resonance imaging of the brain. Atrophic changes of the auditory cortex are observed in both hemispheres

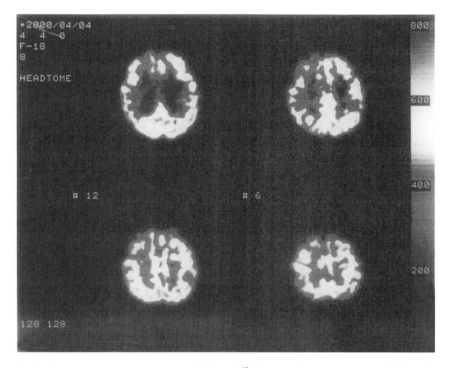

Fig. 4. Positron emission tomography (PET) with ^{18}F-2-fluoro-2 deoxy-D-glucose. PET studies demonstrate a greater decrease in glucose uptake in the right hemisphere than in the left hemisphere

frontotemporoparietal area in both hemispheres, although the decrease was more prominent in the right hemisphere than in the left hemisphere.

Comment

The patient had no history of a CVA but manifested signs of progressive auditory and articulatory disorders, and finally loss of any useful speech or hearing. Because of these problems, communication was not possible among family members except by writing and reading. She had no other neurological problems. Brain MRI did not demonstrate extensive abnormalities of the brain except atrophy of the auditory cortex and Wernicke's area, and PET suggested a decrease in the uptake of glucose in areas around the Sylvian fissures in both hemispheres, including the primary auditory cortex and Wernicke's and Broca's language centers. Neurologically, the patient was suspected to have primary progressive aphasia (PPA) due to frontotemporal dementia (FTD). Her present manifestations appear to be those seen at the early stage of PPA/FTD (6–9). However, a final diagnosis is not possible without her brain being examined neuropathologically.

Provisionally, this patient was diagnosed as having PPA, the onset of which was characterized by cortical deafness and articulatory disorder. This PPA is a type of FTD. FTD encompasses Pick's disease, PPA, and meaning dementia (dementia characterized by the inability to grasp the meaning of spoken words). In conclusion, this rare condition of cortical deafness and anarthria is believed to be an early neurological sign of PPA, and the patient's condition is expected to worsen in the near future.

References

1. Wernicke C, Friedländer C (1883) Ein fall von Taubbeit in folge von doppelseitiger läsion des Schläfelappens. Fortscshr Med 1:6
2. Kaga K, Shindo M, Tanaka Y (1997) Central auditory information processing in patients with bilateral auditory cortex lesions. Acta Otolaryngol (Stockh) Suppl 532:77–82
3. Kaga K, Shindo M, Tanaka Y, et al (2000) Neuropathology of auditory agnosia following bilateral temporal lobe lesions: Acta Otolaryngol 120:259–262
4. Kaga M, Shindo M, Kaga K (2000) Long-term follow-up of auditory agnosia as a sequel of herpes encephalitis in a child. J Child Neurol 15:62–629
5. Kaga K, Yasui T, Yuge F, et al (2003) Auditory agnosia in children after herpes encephalitis. Acta Otolaryngol 123:232–235
6. Kertesz A, Martinez-Lage P, Davidson W, et al (2000) The corticobasal degeneration syndrome overlaps progressive aphasia and frontotemporal dementia. Neurology 55:1368–1375
7. Hodges JR (2001) Frontotemporal dementia (Picke's disease): clinical features and assessment. Neurology 56:s6–s10
8. Essig M, Schroder J (2001) Frontotemporal dementia: clinical neuroimaging and molecular biological findings in six patients. Eur Arch Psychiatr Clin Neurosci 251:225–231
9. Benke T, Donnemiller E (2002) The diagnosis of frontotemporal dementia. Fortschr Neurol Psychiatrie 70:243–251

8
Auditory Agnosia in Children

Auditory Agnosia in Children after Herpes Encephalitis[1]

The mechanism of hearing loss in patients with bilateral auditory cortex lesions remains controversial. This manifestation is known as auditory agnosia or cortical deafness and in adult patients is usually caused by two episodes of cerebral infarction. However, in pediatric cases, it is frequently caused by herpes encephalitis (1–4), not by a cerebrovascular accident (CVA). Adult cases have been extensively studied but pediatric cases have rarely been reported because the residual hearing of these patients is not well documented from developmental and educational standpoints. We report here the cases of four children with auditory agnosia after herpes encephalitis that were studied from neurotological, neuropsychological, and educational standpoints to determine their differences from adult cases.

Case Reports

Four pediatric patients whose bilateral auditory cortices were damaged by herpes encephalitis at an early age were studied. Their brain computed tomography (CT) and magnetic resonance imaging (MRI) scans demonstrated common bilateral lesions of the auditory cortices (Fig. 1). Their auditory perception was investigated by means of behavioral and objective hearing tests and auditory perception tests. All four patients showed mild or moderate hearing loss in the behavioral hearing test (Fig. 2) and normal auditory brainstem responses (ABRs) (Fig. 3), but they did not manifest total deafness. Moreover, perception tests involving speech,

---

[1]This section of the chapter was excerpted from: Kaga K, Kaga M, Tamai F, Shindo M. Auditory agnosia in children after herpes encephalitis. *Acta Otolaryngol* 123:232–235, 2003.

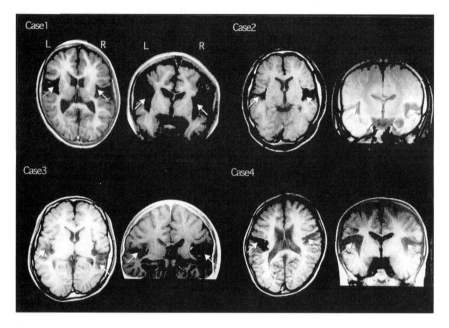

Fig. 1. Brain magnetic resonance scans of the four cases after herpes encephalitis. Note the bilateral lesions (*arrows*) in the superior temporal gyrus, including the auditory cortex

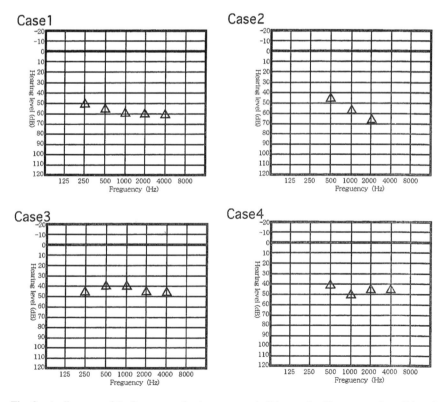

Fig. 2. Audiograms of the four cases after herpes encephalitis examined by means of conditioned orientation reflex audiometry because pure-tone audiometry was difficult. Note the threshold elevation compared to that of age-matched controls

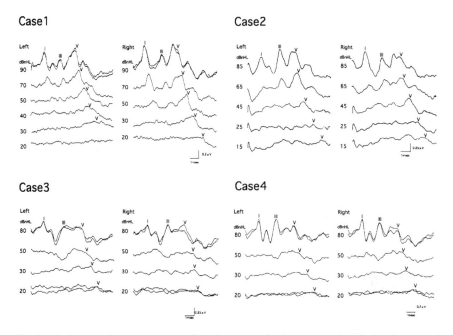

Fig. 3. Auditory brainstem responses of the four cases after herpes encephalitis showing normal configurations and thresholds

environmental sounds, and music demonstrated that most auditory perception ability had been lost in all four patients. On reaching school age, the patients were enrolled in schools for the deaf or special schools for handicapped children.

Comments

Well-known underlying diseases associated with auditory agnosia in children include Landau-Kleffner syndrome and CVAs, such as with moyamoya disease. However, because of the extremely low incidence of auditory agnosia in children, little interest has been paid to it and its manifestations may often go undiagnosed. Auditory agnosia as a sequelae of herpes simplex encephalitis has only recently been discussed (4). Herpes simplex encephalitis is known to lead to focal brain necrosis, particularly in the temporal orbitofrontal regions of the brain. However, reports of language-related sequelae in children caused by focal brain lesions are limited.

Our four patients, having being diagnosed with herpes encephalitis, showed common bilateral temporal lesions of the auditory cortices, which indicated typical auditory agnosia. The early onset of auditory agnosia made their education difficult. Three of the patients went to schools for the deaf, and one was educated at a school for handicapped children. Although their audiograms showed residual hearing, they could not hear in practice. Today all of the patients can read and write Japanese characters, although not perfectly. Because of slow development of the concept of grammar, they experienced difficulty communicating effectively with others. Written communication is almost impossible, despite some writing ability. However, sign language is extremely useful as a communication tool.

Finally, we emphasize that, owing to auditory agnosia, our pediatric patients showed a profound communication disorder. Their present handicaps, despite early, intensive, continuous training, suggest that a more fundamental language deficit is likely to occur in the developing brain than in the mature brain. The communication training and education of these patients can lead to some, but not total, improvement in their communication ability. In the present educational setting, schools for the deaf are better than other schools because they cater to children with such rare disorders as this one who require special education.

References

1. Sugimoto T, Woo M, Okazaki H (1985) Computed tomography in young children with herpes simplex virus encephalitis. Pediatr Radiol 15:372–376
2. Kapur N, Barker S, Burrows EH (1994) Herpes simplex encephalitis: longs-term magnetic resonance imaging and neuropsychological profile. J Neurol Neurosurg Psychiatry 57:1334–1342
3. Ku A, Lachmann EA, Nagler W (1966) Selective language aphasia form herpes simplex encephalitis. Pediatr Neurol 15:169–171
4. Kaga M, Shingo M, Kaga K (2000) Long-term follow-up of auditory agnosia as a sequel of herpes encephalitis in a child. J Child Neurol 15:626–629

Hypogenesis of Cerebral Hemispheres of Infants[2]

The aim of this study was to determine whether cerebral hemispheres are essential for hearing in the presence of a brain anomaly. There are several types of cerebral cortex hypogenesis: hydranencephaly, first described by Crueilher, is a rare and severe anomaly of the central nervous system (CNS) in infants whose entire cerebral hemispheres are nearly destroyed due to vascular disturbances (1). A fluid-filled membranous sac resembling a large cyst mostly replaces the brain. The cause of hydranencephaly is thought to be an occlusive disease of the supraclinoid

---

[2]This section of the chapter was excerpted from: Kaga K, Yasui T, Yuge T. Auditory behaviors and auditory brainstem responses of infants with hypogenesis of cerebral hemispheres. *Acta Otolaryngol* 122:16–20, 2002.

part of the internal carotid artery (1–4), which occurs any time between the third month of gestation and the second postnatal year. It is an important issue with respect to auditory function whether children with a completely absent cerebral cortex but with a preserved brainstem and thalamus are able to hear. If they can hear certain sounds, how should the pathophysiology be considered?

Case Reports

Case 1

A 3-month-old boy had been born after 40 weeks' gestation with no apparent complications during labor or delivery. The Apgar score was 10, and the sucking and Moro reflexes were slightly depressed. His weight at birth was 3.4 kg, head circumference 37 cm, and height 53 cm. His head grew extremely large, and the sunset phenomenon occurred often.

The MRI of the brain revealed that the patient had a brainstem, cerebellum, and thalamus but no cerebral hemispheres, which were replaced by membranous sacs containing cerebrospinal fluid (CSF) (Fig. 1). These findings indicated a rare form of hydranencephaly (i.e., hydrocephalus), which is associated with severe brain malformation.

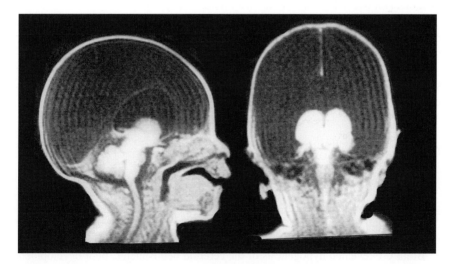

Fig. 1. Brain magnetic resonance imaging (MRI) scans of the patient at 3 months showing the absence of auditory cortices of both bilateral hemispheres

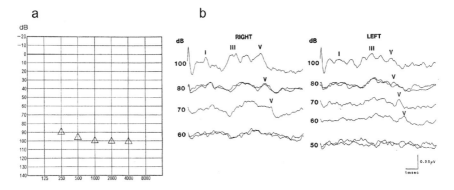

Fig. 2. Patient 1. **a** Behavioral audiometry. **b** Auditory brainstem responses (ABRs) at 3 months

Behavioral audiometry showed responses at 90–100 dB. ABRs showed normal waveforms for both ears at loud click stimulation and a mild threshold elevation (70 dB). However, middle-latency responses (MLRs) and slow vertex responses (SVRs) were absent in both ears (Fig. 2).

Case 2

A 4-year-old boy had been born after 36 weeks' gestation. Because he manifested respiratory distress he was treated with high-pressure oxygen therapy for the first 2 months and was diagnosed with hydranencephaly at 4 months. The sunset phenomenon occurred, and the Babinski reflex was positive.

T2-weighted MRI revealed that the cerebral hemispheres and cerebellum were replaced by CSF and separated by several sacs, but the brainstem was clearly observed (Fig. 3).

Behavioral audiometry showed responses at 48 dB to various frequencies. ABRs showed normal configuration for both ears following stimulation with loud clicks and mild threshold elevation at 25 dB (Fig. 4).

Case 3

An 8-year-old boy had been born following normal labor and delivery at 39 weeks' gestation. His weight at birth was 3.5 kg. Development of motor functions was delayed. Head control and a stable sitting position have not been attained at the present age of 8 years.

Brain CT revealed hypogenesis of the cerebral hemispheres, poor development of the cerebral lobes, but normal development of the brainstem and cerebellum. These findings revealed a totally anterior brain cyst (Fig. 5).

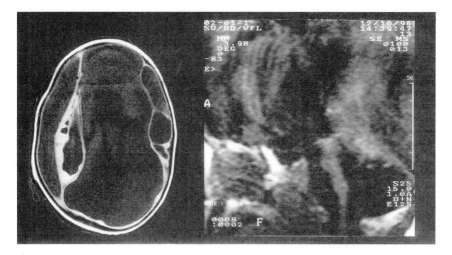

Fig. 3. Patient 2. Brain MRI scan. Bilateral cerebral hemispheres and the cerebellum, which contains numerous cysts, are almost entirely replaced by cerebrospinal fluid

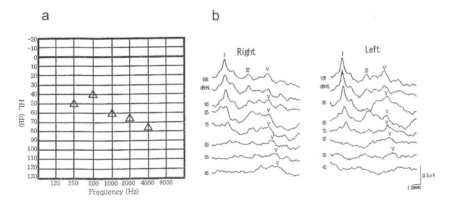

Fig. 4. Patient 2. **a** Behavioral audiometry at 3 years. **b** ABRs at 4 years

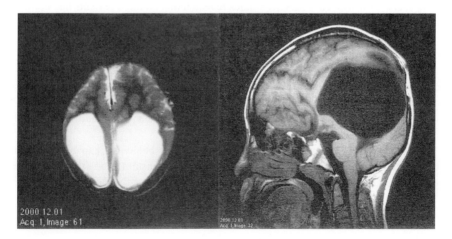

Fig. 5. Patient 3. Brain MRI. Most of the cerebral hemisphere, with the exception of the frontal lobes, is absent, whereas the cerebellum and brainstem are preserved

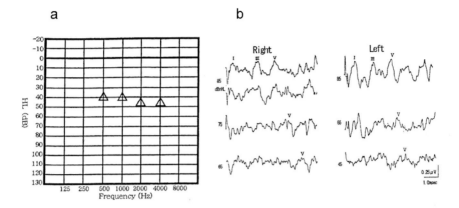

Fig. 6. **a** Patient 3. Behavioral audiometry. **b** ABRs at 5 years

Behavioral audiometry showed responses at 40–45 dB. ABRs had a normal wave configuration following stimulation with loud clicks at 85 dB and a moderate threshold elevation at 65 dB (Fig. 6).

Comment

The MRI and CT investigations of the brains revealed that although these three patients had a brainstem, cerebellum, and thalamus there was an almost complete absence of the cerebral hemispheres, which were replaced by membranous sacs containing CSF. These findings indicated an anomalous form of hydranencephaly (i.e., hydrocephalus), which is associated with severe brain malformations (5–7). Thresholds of behavioral audiometry were 90–100 dB for case 1, 40–80 dB for case 2, and 65 dB for case 3. ABR studies revealed that all three patients had normal wave configurations at loud click stimulation. These findings suggest that behavioral auditory responses can exist in humans if the brainstem structure is preserved, even in the absence of cerebral hemispheres.

Auditory functions and perceptual and cognitive abilities in humans are associated with the cerebral cortex, whereas reflexive behavior originates in the brainstem and midbrain. In neonates and children, auditory functions are measured by behavioral audiometry, conditioned orientation reflex audiometry, play audiometry, and pure-tone audiometry.

Our study reveals that apparent auditory response behaviors can be observed using behavioral audiometry so long as the brainstem and thalamus are preserved.

References

1. Hamby WB, Krauss RF, Beswick WF (1950) Hydranencephaly: clinical diagnosis. Pediatrics 6:371–383
2. Halsey JH, Allen N (1971) The morphogenesis of hydranencephaly. J Neurosci 12:187–217
3. Hanigan WC, Aldrich WM (1988) MRI and evoked potential in a child with hydranencephaly. Pediatr Neurol 4:185–187
4. Mori K, Simada J (1995) Classification of hydrocephalus and outcome of treatment. Brain Dev 17:338–348
5. Nau HE, Reinhardt V (1979) Hydranencephaly: clinical and neuropathological aspects. Acta Neurochir (Wien) 47:219–233
6. Lindberg R, Swanson PD (1967) Infantile hydranencephaly: a report of five cases of infarction of both cerebral hemispheres in infancy. Brain 90:839–850
7. Kaga K, Yasui T, Yuge T (2002) Auditory behaviors and auditory brainstem responses of infants with hypogenesis of cerebral hemispheres. Acta Otolaryngol 122:16–20

Epileptic Auditory Agnosia: Landau-Kleffner Syndrome

Landau-Kleffner syndrome is found with epileptic aphasia syndrome in children with auditory agnosia (1–3). It is caused by epilepsy in the bilateral temporal lobe including the auditory cortex (4). The most important examination is electroencephalography (EEG).

Case Report

We report a case of Landau-Kleffner syndrome with bilateral moderate peripheral hearing loss (Fig. 1). The patient's hearing loss became apparent at age 3 years. ABRs showed a normal (Fig. 2) threshold. She was fitted with a hearing aid and given auditory training. At age 5 years, she suddenly neither responded to speech sounds nor spoke words. She could recognize environmental sounds but not verbal stimuli or melodies. EEG showed bilateral diffuse spike-and-wave complexes (Fig. 3). Although anticonvulsants were prescribed for her, the signs continued and she entered a school for the deaf. At age 7 years she gradually began to speak words again. She is now 13 years old, and the central hearing and inner speech disorders continue. Her auditory comprehension is severely impaired, so she has severe language retardation. We think that her language disorders are caused by both peripheral hearing loss and central auditory and inner speech disorders.

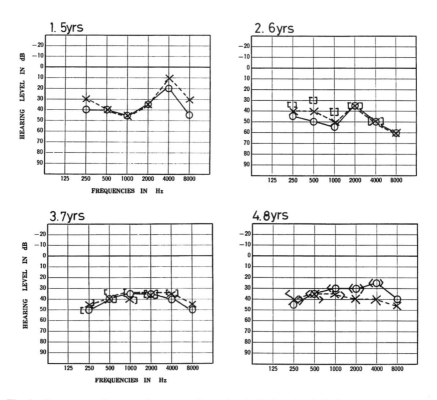

Fig. 1. Pure-tone audiometry shows a moderate threshold elevation in both ears

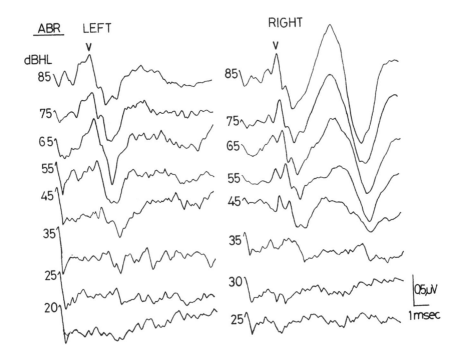

Fig. 2. Auditory brainstem responses (*ABR*) show normal configuration and normal threshold

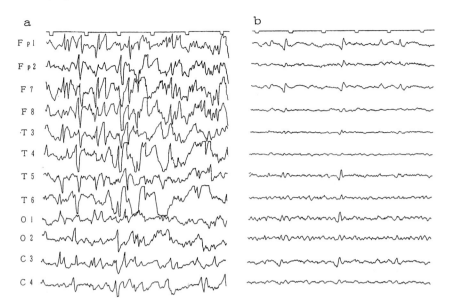

Fig. 3. Electroencephalography findings. **a** At 6 years of age, during the first visit, there is spike-and-wave complex in both hemispheres. **b** At 13 years of age, after administration of anticonvulsants, there are spikes only in the left hemisphere

Comments

There are two theories to account for Landau-Kleffner syndrome. One is selective inhibition of the speech center, and the other is localized inflammation. In the patient manifesting auditory agnosia and epileptic waves in the bilateral temporal lobes, the selective inhibition theory is feasible. It is important to conduct a differential diagnosis using EEG. Anticonvulsive medication is then chosen to control the disease.

Language disorders in Landau-Kleffner syndrome have been reported as symptoms of acquired aphasia, verbal auditory agnosia, or epileptic aphasia. Rapin et al.'s proposal of "verbal auditory agnosia" in 1977 is most often used to describe the main symptoms in Landau-Kleffner syndrome (5).

Regarding the relevant terminology, there has been some confusion in the area of central auditory processing and internal language disorders. For example, auditory agnosia itself is the same as cortical deafness in a wide sense and is the same as auditory verbal agnosia in a narrow sense. Moreover, auditory verbal agnosia is sometimes described as pure word deafness.

Patients with Landau-Kleffner syndrome showed continuous, sequential, and sometimes hierarchical language disorders of sensory aphasia, auditory nonverbal agnosia, and auditory verbal agnosia (word deafness), with or without agnosognosia, during disease progression (4). It is inappropriate to express the language disorder in this syndrome simply as "auditory verbal agnosia."

References

1. Landau WM, Kleffner FR (1957) Syndrome of acquired aphasia with convulsive disorder in children. Neurology (Minneap) 7:523–530
2. Bishop DVM (1985) Age of onset and outcome in "acquired aphasia with convulsive disorder" (Landau-Kleffner syndrome). Dev Med Child Neurol 27:705–712
3. Worster-Drought C (1971) An unusual form of acquired aphasia in children. Dev Med Child Neurol 13:563–571
4. Kaga M (1999) Language disorders in Landau-Kleffner syndrome. J Child Neurol 14:108–122
5. Rapin I, Mattis S, Rowen AJ, et al (1977) Verbal auditory agnosia in children. Dev Med Child Neurol 19:192–207

9
Auditory Cortex Lesion and Sound Lateralization: Interaural Time Difference Versus the Interaural Intensity Difference[1]

Introduction

Sound localization in the horizontal plane primarily depends on the interaural time difference (ITD) and interaural intensity difference (IID). Single-unit techniques have shown that binaural neurons in the auditory cortex of cats (6, 7) are sensitive to the ITD or IID. If identical sounds with the ITD or IID are presented to both ears through earphones, the sound images are lateralized to the side receiving the earlier, or louder, stimulus within the head. The perceptual effects are therefore termed sound lateralization rather than sound localization. In free-field, these two cues are combined with spectral cues provided by the outer ears to characterize the origin of a sound source.

Among patients with unilateral lesions, some studies have shown impairment in localizing sound in the auditory hemi-field contralateral to the damaged hemisphere (1, 2), whereas others have been unable to demonstrate localization deficits in either the ipsilateral or the contralateral auditory hemi-field (3). Contradictory results were also demonstrated in patients with bilateral lesions—i.e., impaired (2, 4) or almost normal (5) ability to localize sound in space.

In patients with temporal lobe lesions, there have been many reports of sound localization in free-field, but dichotic studies of ITD or IID discrimination are rare (8, 9). Moreover, these reports investigated only ITD (8) or only IID (9) discrimination. Thus, the role of the human auditory cortex in discriminating ITD or IID is still not clear.

In the present study, we examined sound lateralizing abilities of patients with left unilateral lesions or bilateral lesions that included the auditory cortex and investigated the role of the auditory cortex in discriminating ITD or IID separately.

[1]The material in this chapter was excerpted from: Yamada K, Kaga K, Uno A, Shindo M (1995) Sound lateralization in patients with lesions including the auditory cortex: comparison of interaural time difference (ITD) discrimination and interaural intensity difference (IID) discrimination. *Hear Res* 101:173–180, 1995; Yamada K, Kaga K, Uno A, Shindo M (1997) Comparison of interaural time and intensity difference discrimination in patients with temporal lobe lesions. Acta Otolaryngol Suppl 532:135–137.

Case Studies

Subjects were 15 patients who had had a cerebrovascular accident (CVA) with lesions that included the auditory cortex (the anterior and posterior transverse temporal gyri of Heschl). They consisted of 12 patients with left unilateral hemispheric lesions and 3 patients with bilateral hemispheric lesions (Table 1). The lesions were confirmed by horizontal and frontal sections of computed tomography (CT) or magnetic resonance imaging (MRI). Clinically, the patients were diagnosed with perceptual disorders of verbal sounds (left unilateral lesions) or auditory agnosia (bilateral lesions) and were in a chronic state—more than 6 months after the CVA—without attentional or intellectual disorders.

All patients could understand what the experimenters wrote (good reading comprehension). In all patients, auditory thresholds for pure tones of 500 Hz were less than 40 dB HL (hearing level), and binaural threshold differences were less than 10 dB (Table 1). In all patients, auditory brainstem responses (ABRs) with 90 dB hearing level (HL) click stimuli did not show any abnormalities. Data from 30 subjects with normal hearing (age 20–58 years; 15 men, 15 women) were used as the control.

The ITD and IID discrimination abilities were separately measured by a self-recording apparatus (TD-01; Rion, Tokyo, Japan) (Fig. 1). This apparatus delivered

Table 1. Patients and ITD and IID discrimination thresholds

Patient	Age (years)	Sex	Lesion site	Auditory threshold (dB) Right	Left	Stimulation level (dB) Right	Left	Discrimination threshold ITD (μs)	IID (dB)
1	35	M	Left	20	20	60	60	402	12.50
2	47	M	Left	5	10	45	50	344	8.25
3	48	F	Left	5	10	45	45	510	
4	52	M	Left	15	15	55	55	536	12.55
5	54	M	Left	15	10	50	50	316	ND
6	55	M	Left	10	5	45	40	292	5.80
7	55	M	Left	15	20	45	55	370	9.70
8	58	M	Left	25	25	65	65	428	9.65
9	60	M	Left	20	25	60	65	424	9.35
10	61	M	Left	35	35	70	70	846	10.70
11	69	F	Left	20	25	50	60	255	ND
12	67	M	Left	20	20	55	55	306	6.65
13	15	M	Bil.	20	30	55	65	—	10.50
14	47	M	Bil.	40	35	70	70	—	
15	63	M	Bil.	30	40	70	75	—	25.94

Auditory threshold, normal hearing level for pure tone at 500 Hz; stimulation level, normal hearing level for noise delivered from each earphone that each patient perceived the sound image at the center of the head
—, off the scale; ND, did not perform the test
ITD, interaural time difference; IID, interaural intensity difference

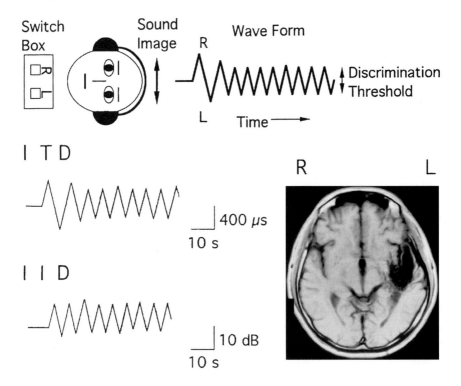

Fig. 1. Schema of the sound lateralization test, the wave form, and the discrimination threshold. Wave form ITD and IID discrimination tests and MRI in a patient with left temporal lobe lesions. MRI was obtained on a horizontal section through the auditory cortex

identical, continuous, narrow-band noise from each earphone. The center frequency and the bandwidth of the noise were 500 Hz and 75 Hz, respectively. The apparatus could create a time difference between the right and left noise ranging from 2 to 200 μs and could also create an intensity difference between them. The noise signal was digitized by an A/D converter (sampling rate 2 μs) and was divided into two signals. One signal was input in a fixed time delay circuit, and the other was input in a variable time delay circuit that varied 2-μs steps at a constant rate of 50 or 100 μs/s (ΔT/T). These digital signals were converted to analog signals and were sent to each earphone through attenuators. The attenuator could vary the intensity of the signal to the right earphone in continuity at a constant rate of 1.25 or 2.50 dB/s (ΔI/T). By varying the ITD or IID constantly, a subject with normal hearing perceived that a sound image made by dichotic noise presentation moved to the right or the left side in the subject's head. ITD and IID discrimination tests were performed in a soundproof room.

Prior to the test, continuous noise was presented to each ear at 35 dB (in nine patients) or 40 dB (in six patients) above the auditory threshold of each ear for pure tones of 500 Hz. Altogether, 9 of the 15 patients perceived that the sound image was at the center of their heads, and the other 6 patients perceived that the sound image was biased toward the right or the left side. In these 6 patients, we then adjusted the output level to the right earphone by an increment or decrement of 5 dB. As a result of the adjustment, all 6 patients answered that the sound image had shifted to the center. In 30 control subjects, 6 subjects also needed an adjustment by 5 dB. The intensity of the noise used in the test in all patients is shown in Table 1.

The test began with a sound image at the center of each subject's head. Subjects received instructions to press the button in the switch box (Fig. 1) as soon as possible after they perceived whether the location of the sound image was biased toward the right or the left side from the center. When an experimenter pressed the start button in the apparatus, the time or intensity difference between dichotic noises increased at a constant rate. If the right noise preceded (or became louder) gradually, a subject with normal hearing could perceive the sound image as moving toward the right side in the head. The subject then pressed the "right" button, and the sound image immediately began to move in the opposite direction, toward the left. Thereafter, the left noise preceded (or became louder), and the subject could perceive the sound image moving to the left side. When the subject pressed the "left" button, the sound image again began to move in the opposite direction, toward the right (Fig. 1). The recording paper moved at 1 mm/s, and traces of sound locomotion were recorded as saw-toothed waves by repetition of the right and left button operations, like Békésy's audiogram.

The interval between the right and left button operations consisted of three parts: 1) from pressing the "right" button until return of the sound image to the center; 2) from return of the sound image to the center until perception of the biased sound image toward the left (perception time); and 3) from perception of the biased sound image until pressing the "left" button (reaction time). It was difficult to draw a clear distinction between perception time and reaction time. Reaction time was usually much shorter than the perception time; therefore, the amplitude of the saw-toothed wave that was drawn between the right and left button operations almost represented the sensitivity of ITD or IID discrimination. We defined the mean amplitude of 10 consecutive saw-toothed waves as the threshold for ITD or IID discrimination. If a subject who could not discriminate ITD or IID performed this test, the subject would not press buttons. Therefore, the recording pen stopped moving at the edge of the recording paper, and the trace showed a linear line.

Results

Waveforms in ITD and IID Discrimination Tests

Figure 2 shows waveforms of four representative patients. Waveforms in both the ITD and IID discrimination tests for patient 1 (Fig. 2a) were almost symmetrical

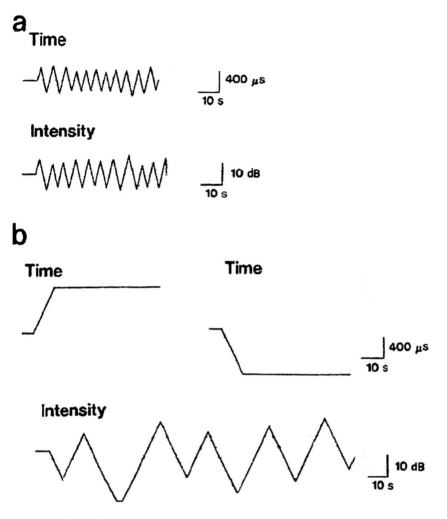

Fig. 2. Waveform from both ITD and IID discrimination tests in two representative patients. **a** Patient 1, normal ITD and IID. **b** Patient 15, ITD shows out of scale and IID reveals remarkable threshold elevation. *Time* indicates the results of the ITD discrimination test. *Intensity* indicates the results of the IID discrimination test

with the midline of the paper, whereas those for patient 8 deviated to the right with time. For patient 2, the waveform in the ITD discrimination test deviated to the left, but the waveform in the IID discrimination test was symmetrical with the midline of the paper. Patient 15 could discriminate IID but not ITD (Fig. 2b).

ITD Discrimination Threshold

In control subjects, ITD thresholds ranged from 92 to 274 μs (mean ± SD: 186.7 ± 50.1 μs). All 12 patients with left unilateral lesions could discriminate ITD. Their ITD thresholds ranged from 244 to 846 μs (mean ± SD 418 ± 160 μs). ITD discrimination thresholds in patients with left unilateral lesions were significantly higher than those in control subjects ($t = 7:16$, $P < 0.01$). None of the three patients with bilateral lesions could discriminate ITD (Table 1).

IID Discrimination Threshold

In control subjects, IID thresholds ranged from 2.9 to 8.7 dB (mean ± SD: 5.5 ± 2.1 dB). In all, 9 of the 12 patients with left unilateral lesions and 2 of the 3 patients with bilateral lesions underwent the IID discrimination test. All of the 11 patients who underwent the IID discrimination test could discriminate IID, but their thresholds were significantly higher than those of the control group ($t = 4.78$, $P < 0.01$). IID discrimination thresholds in patients with left unilateral lesions ranged from 5.80 to 12.55 dB (mean ± SD: 9.46 ± 2.32 dB), and the thresholds in two of the patients with bilateral lesions were 10.50 and 25.94 dB, respectively (Table 1).

All 11 patients who underwent the IID discrimination test could discriminate changes in IID. In the prior test using 5-dB increments to adjust the output level to the right earphone, the remaining four patients with either unilateral or bilateral lesions could also detect where the sound image was (right side, left side, or center of the head). Therefore, the remaining four patients would also have been able to discriminate IID.

Comment

Bisiach et al. (9) investigated sound lateralization using dichotic presentation of pure tones with IID in patients with unilateral damage of the cerebral hemispheres. They found that neither left-brain-damaged patients nor right-brain-damaged patients without any visual field defects showed impairment during this task. In the present study, patients with left unilateral temporal lobe lesions could also discriminate IID.

The IID discrimination thresholds were significantly higher than those in control subjects, and those in patients with bilateral lesions tended to be higher than those in patients with unilateral lesions. This indicated that sensitivity for discriminating IID was reduced when the auditory cortex was damaged. The auditory cortex therefore also plays an important role in discriminating IID. However, results obtained in patients with bilateral lesions in the present study suggested that bilateral auditory cortices were not indispensable for discriminating IID. This was obviously different from discrimination of ITD. The difference between the results of these two tests was also found in patients with lesions in the lower auditory pathway. Using the same apparatus, we previously studied ITD and IID discrimination in patients with lesions in the acoustic nerve or the brainstem. Some of them could not detect the change in ITD, but all patients could discriminate IID (10).

Coding of ITD and IID has been completed at the level of the mammalian medial geniculate body (MGB). Both ITD- and IID-sensitive neurons in the MGB have projection to the auditory cortex, and IID-sensitive neurons may also have projection to other cortices. Therefore, changes in IID may be detected without bilateral auditory cortices. The role of the auditory cortex may not be essential for indiscriminating IID.

Finally, in patients with left unilateral or bilateral auditory cortical lesions, our results indicated that the auditory cortex plays an important role in discriminating both ITD and IID. In fact, it appears to be necessary for discriminating ITD.

References

1. Sanchez-Longo LP, Forster FM (1957) Clinical significance of impairment of sound localization. Neurology 8:119–125
2. Klingon GH, Bontecou DC (1966) Localization in auditory space. Neurology 16:879–886
3. Shankweiler DP (1961) Performance of brain-damaged patients on two tests of sound localization. J Comp Physiol Psychol 54:375–381
4. Jerger J, Weikers NJ, Sharbrough FW III, Jerger S (1969) Bilateral lesions of the temporal lobe: a case study. Acta Otolaryngol (Stockh) 258:S1–S51
5. Jerger J, Lovering L, Wertz M (1972) Auditory disorder following bilateral temporal lobe insult: report of a case. J Speech Hear Dis 37:523–535
6. Hall JL, Goldstein MH Jr (1968) Representation of binaural stimuli by single units in primary auditory cortex of unanesthetized cats. J Acoust Soc Am 43:456–461
7. Kitzes LM, Wrege KS, Cassady JM (1980) Patterns of responses of cortical cells to binaural stimulation. J Comp Neurol 192:455–472
8. Walsh EG (1958) An investigation of sound localization in patients with neurological abnormalities. Brain 80:222–250
9. Bisiach E, Cornacchia L, Sterzi R (1984) Disorders of perceived auditory lateralization after lesions of the right hemisphere. Brain 107:37–52
10. Yamada K, Kaga K (1991) A study on ITD and IID of patients with ABR wave abnormalities due to brainstem damage. Audiol Jpn 34:238–243

10
Corpus Callosum Lesions[1]

The localization and function of auditory fibers in the corpus callosum in humans are still unclear. The corpus callosum is anatomically divided into four segments: rostrum, genu, truncus, and splenium (from anterior to posterior) (Fig. 1). After the introduction of magnetic resonance imaging (MRI), extinction of the left ear by the dichotic listening or speech perception test has been reported with reference to lesions in the corpus callosum (1–4).

It is important to assess cognitive functions objectively utilizing neurophysiological testing, including P300 event-related potentials in patients with callosal section because their auditory information is processed independently in separate hemispheres. The purpose of this study was twofold: one aim was to elucidate the segment of the corpus callosum responsible for auditory information processing between the two hemispheres; the other aim was to identify the auditory modalities that are processed across the corpus callosum using the modified method of P300 potentials, including pure-tone, monosyllable, and spoken-word stimuli in a patient with callosal section.

Case Report

A 46-year-old right-handed woman complained of dizziness and transient right hemiparesis in March 1988. Computed tomography (CT) revealed a large calcified meningioma in the right lateral ventricle. In May 1988, she underwent extirpation of this tumor, and during the operation the truncus of the corpus callosum was sectioned. Postoperative MRI showed that the posterior portion of the corpus callosum was clearly sectioned with the anterior commissure and splenium

[1]The material in this chapter was excerpted from: Kaga K, Shindo M, Gotho O, Tamaru A (1990) Speech perception and auditory P300 potentials after section of the posterior half of the truncus of the corpus callosum. *Brain Topography* 3:175–181, 1990.

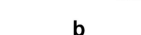

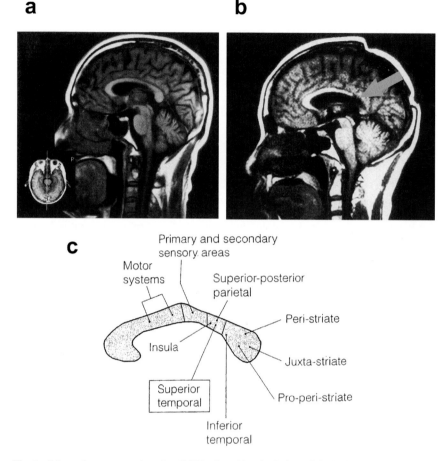

Fig. 1. Magnetic resonance imaging (MRI) of a midsagittal view of the brain. **a** Normal subject. **b** Postoperative MRI of a patient. **c** Midsagittal view shows a section of anterior genu and the posterior truncus of the corpus callosum

spared (Fig. 1). Postoperatively, the patient did not manifest any audiological symptoms or neurological signs, but she complained of mild discomfort in the left ear.

Audiological Testing

A combination of conventional pure-tone audiometry, the 100-monosyllable perception test that was developed by our group, and dichotic listening for three pairs of digits recorded on the tape, was carried out in a soundproof room. The computer-

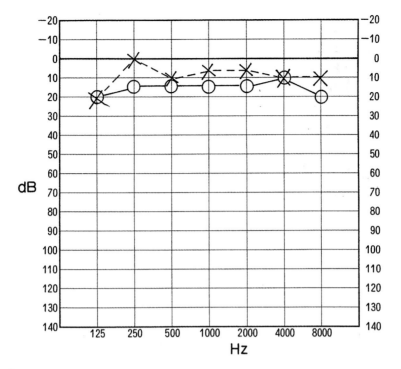

Fig. 2. Pure-tone and speech audiometry. There is no right–left difference

ized sound lateralization test developed by Dr. T. Saito (Tokyo Metropolitan Police Hospital) was also performed; the sound stimuli within a 500-Hz band were produced with differences in time (duration) or loudness (intensity) and moved automatically between the right and left ears.

- Pure-tone audiometry—There was a normal range of thresholds for each frequency in both ears (Fig. 2).
- 100-Monosyllable perception test—The percentage of correct responses in the right ear (92%) was greater than that in the left ear (82%), the difference being approximately 10%. By the unpaired t-test, this right–left difference was considered statistically significant when compared with the normal controls (Fig. 3a).
- Dichotic listening test—The percentage of correct responses in the right ear (97%) was strikingly greater than that in the left ear (12%) (Fig. 3b). This right–left difference suggests that extinction in the left ear occurred under the competitive situation between two ears owing to the callosal section. Regarding this result, it is emphasized that all stimuli were correctly reported for both ears by the patient.
- Sound lateralization test—There were no abnormalities in the interaural time difference or the interaural intensity difference.
- Word recognition test—There was no right–left difference in the results of this test.

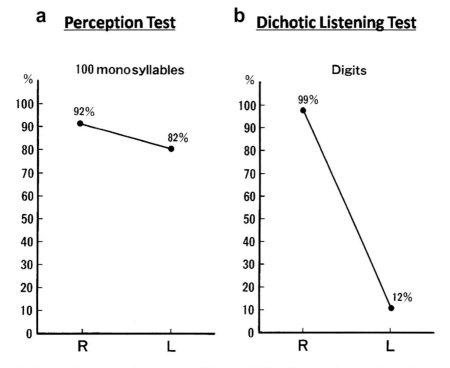

Fig. 3. **a** Auditory perception test using 100 monosyllables. The score for the left ear is lower than that for the right ear. **b** Dichotic listening test. There is a large difference between the right and left ears

Neurophysiological Testing

- Exogenous auditory evoked potentials—Auditory brainstem, middle-latency, and slow vertex responses were all elicited well without an obvious right–left difference. The threshold of the auditory brainstem responses (ABRs) was 20 dB in both ears.
- Endogenous evoked potentials, P300—The results of the P300 testing for each stimulus were visually inspected by three independent examiners and the waveforms for rare and frequent stimuli were compared for each type of acoustic stimulus. Figure 4 shows the P300 potentials to pure tones (1 and 2 kHz) for each ear. The top figures in Fig. 4 were obtained from the first session (I), and the bottom figures from the second session (II). The rare and frequent stimuli were reversed for the second session. The difference between rare and frequent stimuli is obtained by subtracting the waveform for the frequent stimuli from that of the rare stimuli. The shaded areas indicate the rare–frequent difference in the positivity between 300 and 500 ms that may correspond to the P300 potential. Large P300 potentials were observed for the rare pure-tone and word stimuli.

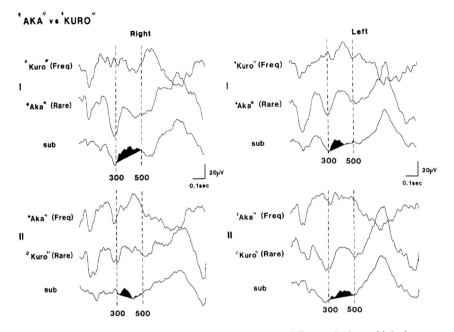

Fig. 4. P300 potentials for spoken-word stimuli. There was a difference in the positivity between 300 and 500 ms. Larger positive potentials were seen for the rare stimuli during each session. Word stimuli: *Aka* means red, and *Kuro* means black. *I, II*, first and second sessions; *sub*, difference between rare and frequent (*Freq.*) stimuli; *shaded areas*, rare–frequent difference in positivity between 300 and 500 ms, possibly corresponding to the P300 potential

Comment

Pendya et al. (5) traced callosal auditory fibers in rhesus monkeys, but there is little specific information about the topography of callosal auditory pathways in humans. A limited number of patients with complete callosal section have been evaluated for callosal auditory function since Sparks and Geschwind (1) showed by dichotic techniques that complete auditory extinction to stimuli (digits or names of animals) presented to the left ear was associated with callosal section. Springer and Gazzaniga (2) demonstrated that left ear extinction was associated with callosal section anterior to the splenium but posterior to the first one-third of the callosum.

In the present case, after section of the posterior half of the truncus of the corpus callosum, striking left-ear extinction was seen for monosyllables in the dichotic listening test, and a mild left-ear deficit was observed for monosyllables in the monaural perception test. In the literature (1–4), most of the patients who showed left-ear extinction had lesions in the posterior half of the truncus or upper splenium of the corpus callosum, as seen in the present case. These findings suggest that the auditory fibers may pass across the posterior body of the corpus callosum in humans, as in the rhesus monkey.

Speech information from the right ear is conveyed to the left auditory cortex near Wernicke's area after crossing over at the level of the superior olivary complex and is then perceived. In addition, speech information from the left ear is transmitted to the left auditory cortex after running through the right auditory cortex and auditory callosal fibers. Because of these anatomical pathways, the discrimination for monosyllables by the right ear is mildly impaired when the left auditory cortex is damaged, and function of the left ear is slightly impaired when the right auditory cortex is damaged; this phenomenon is called a "lesion effect." On the other hand, the right-ear advantage in the dichotic listening test seen in right-handed subjects is called a "dominance effect." In the present case, both lesion and dominance effects seemed to produce left-ear extinction, which appeared mildly in the monosyllable perception test and markedly in the dichotic listening test but did not appear with pure-tone audiometry or the word recognition task. Similar results were observed in studies of the P300 potential, as P300 potentials to the monosyllabic stimuli were absent but those to pure-tone and spoken-word stimuli were well performed.

Our findings suggest that section of the posterior half of the truncus of the corpus callosum results in a difference in stimulus discrimination of the P300 paradigm and in speech discrimination; thus, P300 could be a sensitive indicator of information-processing functions in these patients. Finally, the P300 potential may prove useful in clarifying the nature of cognitive function in patients with callosal sectioning.

References

1. Sparks R, Geschwind N (1968) Dichotic listening in man after section of neocortical commissures. Cortex 1:3–16
2. Springer SP, Gazzaniga MS (1975) Dichotic testing of partial and complete split brain subjects. Neuropsychologia 13:341–346
3. Alexander MP, Warren RL (1988) Localization of callosal auditory pathways: a case study. Neurology 38:802–804
4. Musiek EF, Reeves A (1986) Effects of partial and complete corpus callosotomy on central auditory function. In: Sperry RW (ed) Two hemispheres—one brain. Alan R. Liss, New York, pp 423–433
5. Pendya DN, Karol EA, Heilbron D (1971) The topographic distribution of interhemispheric projections in the corpus callosum of the rhesus monkey. Brain Res. 32:31–43

Subject Index